Handbook of
Diabetes
second edition

Gareth Williams MA, MD, FRCP

Professor of Medicine, University of Liverpool;
Honorary Consultant Physician, University Hospital Aintree,
Liverpool, UK

John C. Pickup MA, BM, BCh, DPhil, FRCPath

Reader & Consultant, Division of Chemical Pathology,
Guy's, King's & St Thomas' Hospitals School of Medicine, Guy's Hospital,
London, UK

b

**Blackwell
Science**

To **Caroline, Timothy, Joanna, Sally and Pippa;
Selma, Matthew, Charlotte and Joshua**

© 1992, 1999 by
Blackwell Science Ltd
Editorial Offices:
Osney Mead, Oxford OX2 0EL
25 John Street, London WC1N 2BL
23 Ainslie Place, Edinburgh EH3 6AJ
350 Main Street, Malden
  MA 02148 5018, USA
54 University Street, Carlton
  Victoria 3053, Australia
10, rue Casimir Delavigne
  75006 Paris, France

Other Editorial Offices:
Blackwell Wissenschafts-Verlag GmbH
Kurfürstendamm 57
10707 Berlin, Germany

Blackwell Science KK
MG Kodenmacho Building
7–10 Kodenmacho Nihombashi
Chuo-ku, Tokyo 104, Japan

Iowa State University Press
A Blackwell Science Company
2121 S. State Avenue
Ames, Iowa 50014-8300, USA

First published 1992
Reprinted 1994, 1997
Revised and updated 1998
Second edition 1999
Reprinted 2000
Revised and reprinted 2001, (twice)

Text layout and design by
The Designers Collective Limited
Printed and bound in Great Britain
at the Alden Group, Oxford.

DISTRIBUTORS

Marston Book Services Ltd
PO Box 269
Abingdon, Oxon OX14 4YN
(*Orders*: Tel: 01235 465500
        Fax: 01235 465555)

USA
Blackwell Science, Inc.
350 Main Street,
Malden, MA 02148 5018
(*Orders*: Tel: 800 759 6102
           781 388 8250
        Fax: 781 388 8255)

Canada
Login Brothers Book Company
324 Saulteaux Crescent
Winnipeg, Manitoba R3J 3T2
(*Orders*: Tel: 204 837 2987)

Australia
Blackwell Science Pty Ltd
54 University Street
Carlton, Victoria 3053
(*Orders*: Tel: 3 9347 0300
        Fax: 3 9347 5001)

A catalogue record for this title
is available from the British Library
and the Library of Congress

ISBN 0-632-05504-9

For further information on
Blackwell Science, visit our website:
www.blackwell-science.com

Contents

Preface to the second edition

The first edition of this book, published in 1991, was intended to present a broad picture of diabetes and its care, and to 'unite many different disciplines in the battle against its many problems'. This second edition also hopes to combine practical aims with lofty sentiments and should again—we hope—appeal to a wide range of people concerned with managing diabetes. Indeed, this book should contain something for everyone, including doctors, specialists and general nurses, chiropodists and dieticians, irrespective of whether they work in hospitals, the community, private practice or a shared-care setting. We have not written it primarily for diabetic patients, but some will undoubtedly find it of interest in providing background information to their own management.

As in the first edition, we have deliberately highlighted the 'science' where this is particularly relevant to 'clinical practice'. In general, the boundary between these two aspects of medicine is becoming more and more blurred, and diabetes provides some excellent examples of how quickly advances in 'science' can be applied to improve the routine clinical care of important diseases. One such example is insulin resistance, which has evolved in only a few years from a rather abstract concept to an important and promising target for novel anti-diabetic drugs.

A few glances at the first and second editions will show how much our understanding of diabetes, and our ability to cope with it, have both moved on. The recent advances covered here include the long-awaited findings of the UK Prospective Diabetes Study, the new diagnostic criteria proposed by the American Diabetes Association, and new drugs to treat diabetes and its complications, including insulin analogues and oral hypoglycaemic agents. For those who are inclined towards 'science', there are new sections on the genetic, immune and environmental causes of type 1 diabetes, the aetiology of insulin resistance in type II diabetes, and the biochemistry of chronic diabetic complications.

The same comparative glances will show that the style and presentation of this book have also leapt forward. The layout and design have been completely changed and will, we believe, help to make the book useful as both a rapid reference work in a busy clinic and an accessible source of knowledge for quiet study. The *Handbook* derives ultimately from the second edition of the *Textbook of Diabetes*, which was published in 1997. However, this Handbook is not merely a cut-down version of the *Textbook*, but a carefully designed and updated selection of key information from it. We hope that you'll enjoy it.

Most people who claim to enjoy writing medical books are not being economical with the truth. They are lying. Exceptionally, however, this one was great fun. This is due quite simply to the vast amounts of time, effort and general niceness that have been devoted to this project by a long list of people—to all of whom we owe our heartfelt thanks. First and foremost are the experts from throughout the world who originally contributed the chapters in the second edition of the *Textbook*; the excellence of their work made the task of producing this book so much easier. Secondly, we are immensely grateful to our friends and colleagues at Blackwell Science. The Designers Collective, headed by Mark Willey, have brought forth an extremely original and attractive book, and with this and the *Textbook*, Blackwell Science have managed to prove that both big and small can be beautiful. Also at Blackwell Science, we are indebted to Andrew Robinson, our editor-in-chief, and to Alice Nelson and John Ashworth. Andrew deserves special mention for remaining wise, patient, good natured and in a fair state of repair after working with us for over a decade. Thirdly, Mimi Chen and Colm Owens appeared to enjoy checking the proofs, and showed no mercy in their hounding of errors that we had missed.

Finally, we must thank our wives (still the same ones) and our families for their support and encouragement and—for reasons that none of us can really explain—for allowing us to do this again.

GARETH WILLIAMS
JOHN C PICKUP

Liverpool and London, August 1999

Chapter 1
Introduction to diabetes

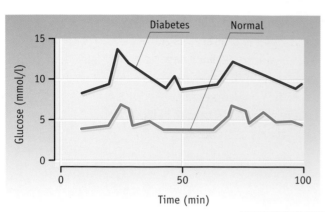

Diabetes mellitus is a condition in which there is a chronically raised blood glucose concentration. It is caused by an absolute or relative lack of the hormone insulin, i.e. insulin is not being produced from the pancreas or there is insufficient insulin or insulin action for the body's needs.

Figure 1.1
Raised blood glucose concentrations in diabetes.

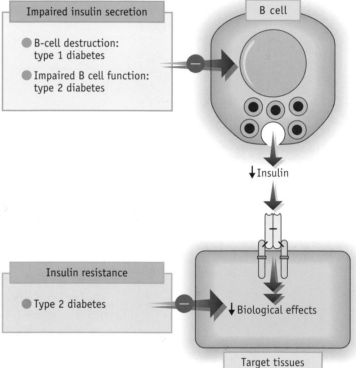

Figure 1.2
Defects in islet B cell and in insulin action in type 1 and 2 diabetes.

The two main types of diabetes are type 1, or insulin-dependent diabetes, and type 2, or non-insulin-dependent diabetes. Type 1 diabetes presents mainly in childhood and early adult life and accounts for about 20% of cases in Europe and North America. It is thought to be caused by an autoimmune destruction of the insulin-producing B cells of the islets of Langerhans.

Figure 1.3
Type 1 diabetes in children or young adults.

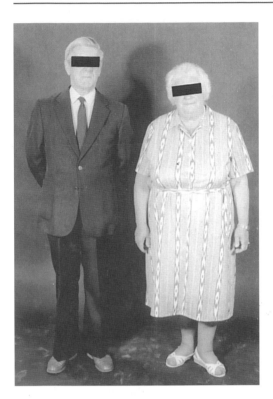

Type 2 diabetes usually starts in middle age or in the elderly. Type 2 diabetes is more common, representing about 80% of cases in most European countries and North America. It is thought to be due to both impaired insulin secretion and resistance to the action of insulin at its target cells. About 80% of type 2 diabetic patients are obese.

Figure 1.4
Lean and obese patients with type 2 diabetes.

Figure 1.5
Diabetic retinopathy, an example of microvascular disease.

One of the most important clinical features of diabetes is its association with chronic tissue complications. These generally occur after several years of diabetes and affect the small blood vessels (microangiopathy) in the eye, kidney and nerves. The frequency of arterial disease (atherosclerosis or macroangiopathy) is also markedly increased. Microangiopathy, at least, is thought to be related to the duration and severity of hyperglycaemia.

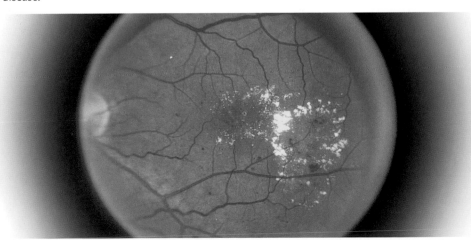

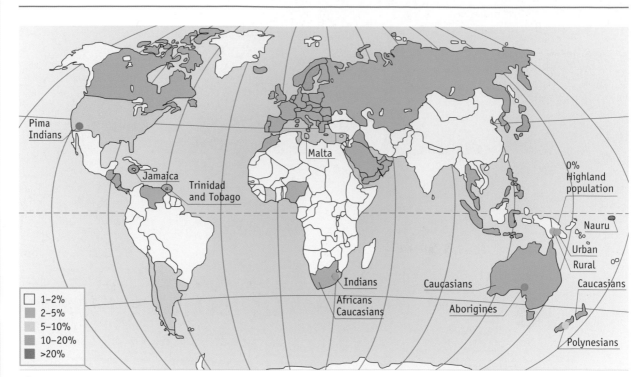

Figure 1.6
The frequency of diabetes throughout the world.

Diabetes is a common disease, with major global public health consequences. In most of Europe about 1–2% of the population suffer from diabetes; in the USA about 3–8% of the white population have diabetes. There are particularly high frequencies in developing countries and ethnic minorities in industrial societies, such as the Pima Indians in the USA and Indian Asians living in the UK. The world prevalence of diabetes is at least 100 million people, a figure which is predicted to double over the next 10–15 years.

Chapter 2
History of diabetes

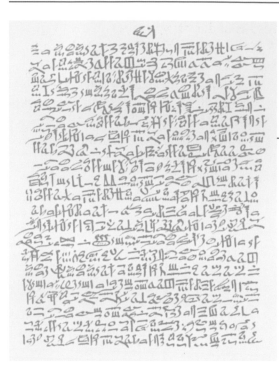

Figure 2.1
The Ebers papyrus.

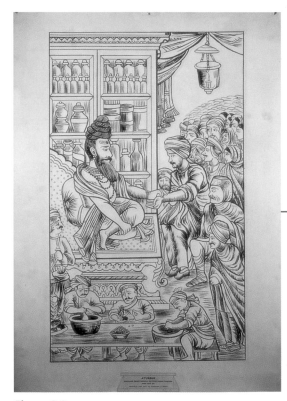

Figure 2.3
Susruta, an Indian physician.

Diabetes has been recognised as a disease since antiquity. The Ebers papyrus dates from 1550 BC and describes a polyuric state resembling diabetes. The papyrus was discovered in 1862 by the German Egyptologist, George Ebers.

The word 'diabetes' comes from the Greek, meaning 'to pass through'. It was first used by Aretaeus of Cappadocia in the 2nd century AD. Aretaeus gave a clinical description of the disease, noting the increased urine flow, thirst and weight loss, features which are instantly recognisable today.

Diabetes is a dreadful affliction, not very frequent among men, being a melting down of the flesh and limbs into urine. The patients never stop making water and the flow is incessant, like the opening of aqueducts. Life is short, unpleasant and painful, thirst unquenchable, drinking excessive, and disproportionate to the large quantity of urine, for yet more urine is passed. One cannot stop them either from drinking or making water. If for a while they abstain from drinking, their mouths become parched and their bodies dry; the viscera seem scorched up, the patients are affected by nausea, restlessness and a burning thirst, and within a short time, they expire.

Figure 2.2
Description of diabetes by Aretaeus.

The sweet, honey-like taste of urine in polyuric patients, which attracted ants and other insects, was reported during the 5th and 6th century AD by Indian physicians such as Susruta. These descriptions even mention two forms of diabetes, one in older, fatter people and the other in thin people who do not survive for long. This division predicted the modern classification into type 2 and type 1 diabetes.

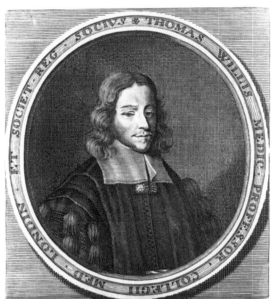

Figure 2.4
Thomas Willis.

The sweetness of diabetic urine was rediscovered in the 17th century by the English physician, Thomas Willis (1621–1675). Willis, who was King Charles II's physician, also remarked that, although the disease was rare in ancient times, its frequency was increasing in his time 'given to good fellowship and gusling down chiefly of unallayed wine'. Nearly a century later in 1776, the Liverpool physician, Matthew Dobson (1735–1784), showed that the sweetness in both urine and serum was due to sugar.

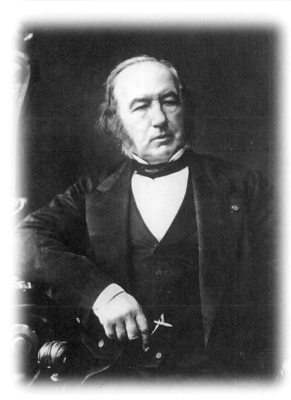

Figure 2.5
Claude Bernard.

The French physiologist, Claude Bernard (1813–1878), made many discoveries in the 19th century relating to diabetes. Amongst these was the finding that sugar appearing in the urine is stored in the liver as glycogen.

Claude Bernard also demonstrated links between the central nervous system and diabetes with his famous 'piqûre diabetes' experiments, where hyperglycaemia was caused by transfixing the medulla of conscious rabbits.

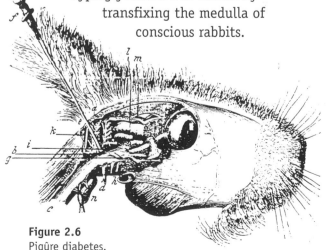

Figure 2.6
Piqûre diabetes.

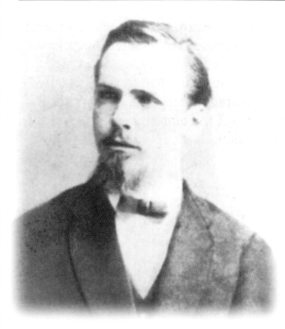

Paul Langerhans (1847–1888) from Berlin was the first to describe, in his 1869 doctoral thesis, small clusters of cells in teased preparations of the pancreas which are now known as the 'islets of Langerhans'. He did not speculate on the function of the cells, and it was Edouard Laguesse in 1893 who named the cells 'islets of Langerhans' and suggested that they were the endocrine tissue of the pancreas.

Figure 2.7
Paul Langerhans.

In 1889, Oskar Minkowski (1858–1931) and Josef von Mering (1849–1908) from Strasbourg removed the pancreas from a dog in order to see if the organ was essential for life. The animal displayed typical signs of diabetes, with thirst, polyuria and wasting, which were associated with glycosuria and hyperglycaemia. This experiment showed that a pancreatic disorder causes diabetes, but they did not follow up this important observation.

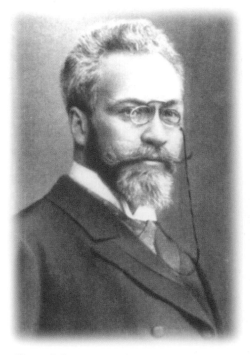

Figure 2.8
Oskar Minkowski.

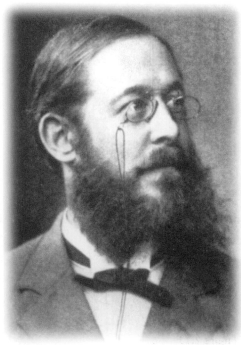

Figure 2.9
Josef von Mering.

HANDBOOK OF DIABETES *2ND EDITION*

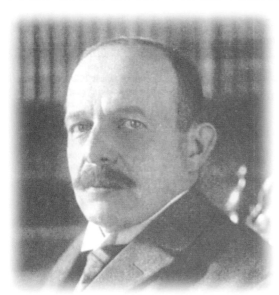

In the early 20th century, various workers isolated impure hypoglycaemic extracts from the pancreas, including the Berlin physician Georg Zuelzer, the Romanian Nicolas Paulesco (1869–1931), and the Americans E.L. Scott and Israel Kleiner. Toxic side-effects were amongst the problems which prevented further investigation.

Figure 2.10
Georg Zuelzer.

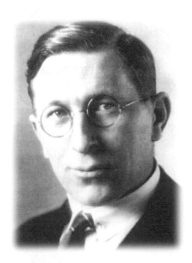
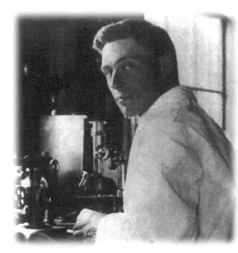
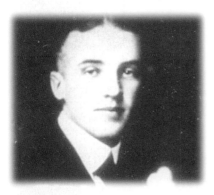
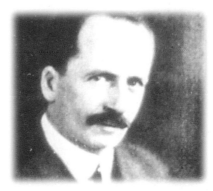

Insulin was discovered at the University of Toronto, Canada, in 1921 through a collaboration between the surgeon Frederick G. Banting (1891–1941), his student assistant Charles H. Best (1899–1978), the biochemist James B. Collip (1892–1965) and the physiologist J.J.R. Macleod (1876–1935).

Figure 2.11
The discoverers of insulin. Clockwise from top left: Frederick G. Banting, James B. Collip, J.J.R. Macleod and Charles H. Best.

Banting and Best made chilled extracts of dog pancreas, injected them into pancreactectomised, diabetic dogs, and showed a decline in blood sugar concentrations.

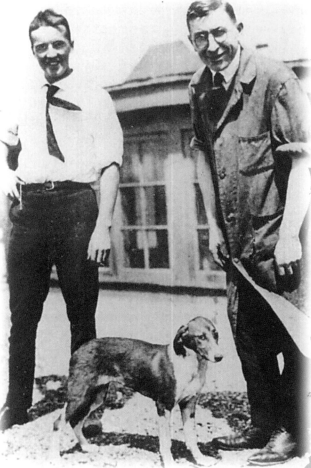

Figure 2.12
Charles Best and Frederick Banting in Toronto in 1922 (the dog is thought to have been called Marjorie).

Banting and Best's notes of the dog experiments refer to the administration of 'isletin', later called 'insulin' by them at the request of Macleod, although this name had already been given to the hormone in 1909 by the Belgian researcher Jean de Meyer.

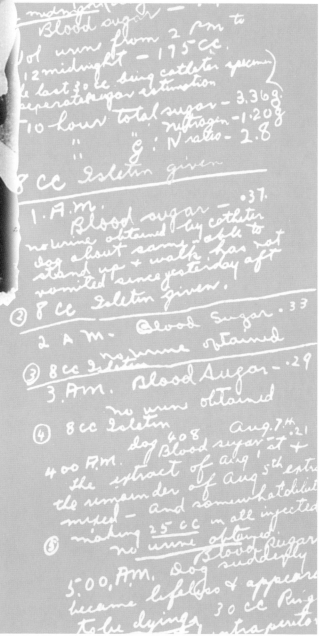

Figure 2.13
Banting and Best's notebook.

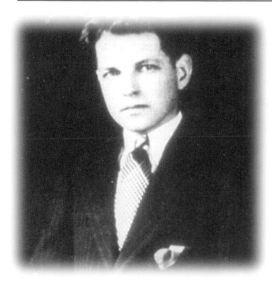

Figure 2.14
Leonard Thompson.

Collip developed an improved extraction and purification procedure and the first diabetic patient, a 14-year-old boy called Leonard Thompson, was treated on 1 January 1922. A commercially viable extraction method was then developed in collaboration with chemists from Eli Lilly and Co. in the USA, and insulin became widely available in North America and Europe from 1923.

The American physician, Elliot P. Joslin was one of the first doctors to gain experience with insulin. Working in Boston, Massachusetts, he treated 293 patients in the first year after August 1922. Joslin also introduced systematic education for his diabetic patients.

Robin B. Lawrence (1892–1968) was an English physician working at King's College Hospital, London. He developed type 1 diabetes shortly before insulin became available and subsequently played a leading part in founding the British Diabetic Association.

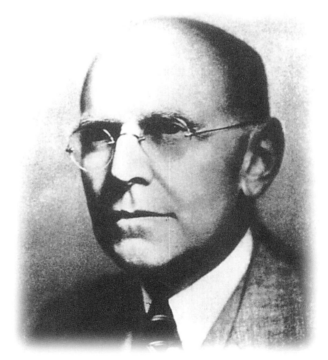

Figure 2.15
Elliot P. Joslin.

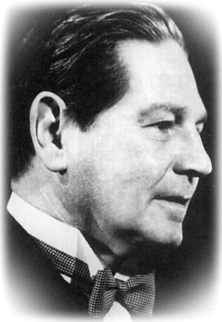

Figure 2.16
Robin B. Lawrence.

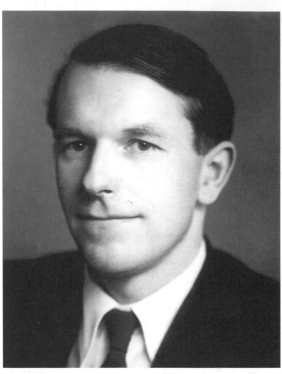

Figure 2.17
Frederick Sanger.

Amongst the many major advances since the introduction of insulin into clinical practice has been the elucidation in 1955, by the Cambridge scientist Frederick Sanger (b. 1918), of the primary structure of insulin, i.e. the amino acid sequence in the two chains of the molecule. Sanger received the Nobel prize for his work in 1958.

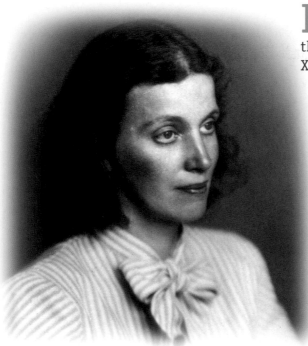

Figure 2.18
Dorothy Hodgkin.

Dorothy Hodgkin (1910–1994), another Nobel prize winner, and her colleagues described the three-dimensional structure of insulin using X-ray crystallography data (1969).

Chapter 3
Diagnosis of diabetes

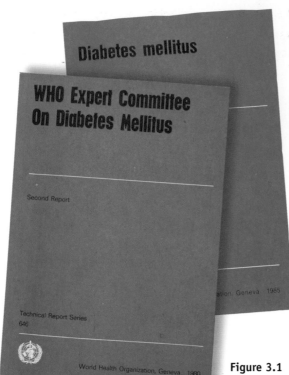

Diabetes is diagnosed by identifying chronic hyperglycaemia. However, until the late 1970s several different diagnostic criteria were applied to the glycaemic response to varying glucose loads, resulting in wide variations in the reported prevalence of diabetes. An international consensus was finally reached with the World Health Organization (WHO) recommendations in 1980 for both the diagnosis and classification of diabetes. These criteria have been widely accepted until 1997, when the American Diabetes Association (ADA) suggested new criteria (see p.17).

Figure 3.1
WHO reports on diabetes.

The WHO diagnostic criteria were based on epidemiological studies of the natural history of glucose intolerance, particularly the level of blood glucose which is associated with microvascular complications such as retinopathy, regarded as the hallmark of diabetes.

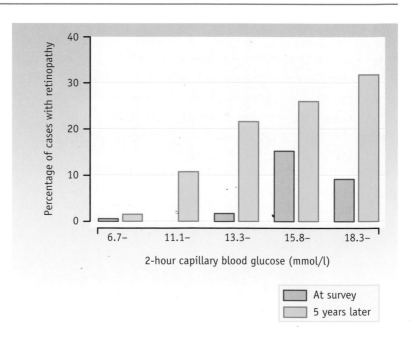

Figure 3.2
Frequency of retinopathy in subjects in the Bedford Survey (R.J. Jarrett, H. Keen) as a function of 2-hour capillary blood level glucose after a 50-g oral glucose load. Retinopathy was seen only in those with blood glucose > about 200 mg/dl (11.1 mmol/l).

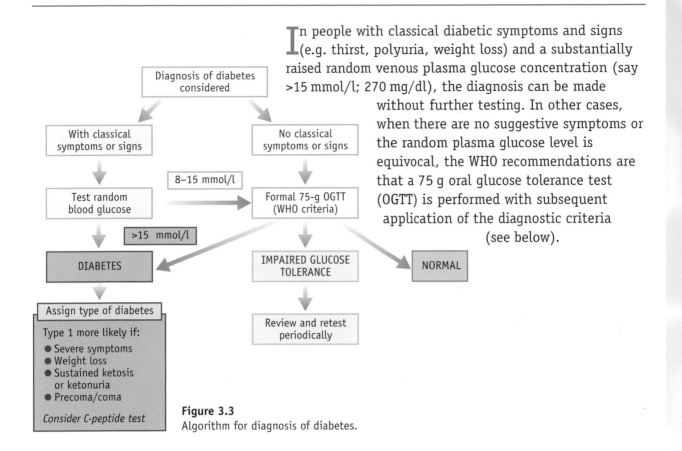

Figure 3.3
Algorithm for diagnosis of diabetes.

In people with classical diabetic symptoms and signs (e.g. thirst, polyuria, weight loss) and a substantially raised random venous plasma glucose concentration (say >15 mmol/l; 270 mg/dl), the diagnosis can be made without further testing. In other cases, when there are no suggestive symptoms or the random plasma glucose level is equivocal, the WHO recommendations are that a 75 g oral glucose tolerance test (OGTT) is performed with subsequent application of the diagnostic criteria (see below).

For the OGTT, the subject is tested in the morning, after an overnight fast, in the seated position, and desisting from smoking. After taking a fasting blood sample, 75 g of glucose is given by mouth, often in the form of a glucose drink such as Lucozade (388 ml). For children, 1.75 g/kg is given. A further blood sample is taken at 2 hours.

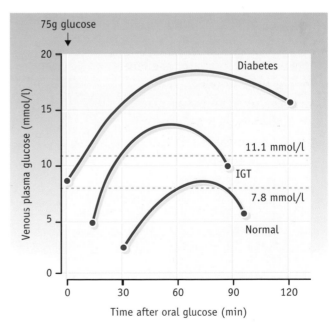

Figure 3.4
Diagnosis of diabetes by the oral glucose tolerance test.
Fasting plasma glucose is >7.8 mmol/l and/or the level exceeds 11.1 mmol/l 2 hours after drinking 75 g of glucose.

Diabetes is diagnosed when the fasting plasma glucose exceeds 7.8 mmol/l (140 mg/dl) and/or the value 2 hours after the glucose load exceeds 11.1 mmol/l (200 mg/dl). The WHO criteria recognises an intermediate zone of abnormal blood glucose levels called 'impaired glucose tolerance' (IGT)—often regarded as kind of borderline diabetes. IGT is diagnosed when the 2-hour glucose value is 7.8–11.1 mmol/l (140–200 mg/dl).

	Glucose concentration in mmol/l (mg/dl)			
	Plasma		Whole blood	
	Venous	Capillary	Venous	Capillary
Diabetes mellitus Fasting value or	≥7.8 (140)	>7.8 (140)	≥6.7 (120)	≥6.7 (120)
2 h after 75 g glucose load	≥11.1 (200)	≥12.2 (220)	≥10.0 (180)	≥11.1 (200)
IGT Fasting value or	<7.8 (140)	<7.8 (140)	<6.7 (120)	<6.7 (120)
2 h after 75 g glucose load	7.8–11.0 (140–199)	8.9–12.1 (160–219)	6.7–9.9 (120–179)	7.8–11.0 (140–199)

Figure 3.5
WHO diagnostic criteria for diabetes and impaired glucose tolerance.

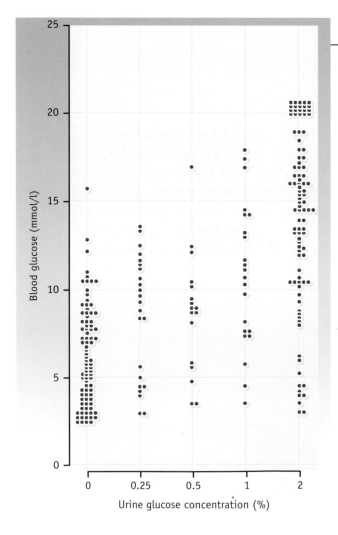

Although the presence of glucose in the urine indicates the need to test blood glucose, glycosuria cannot be used to diagnose diabetes because of the poor relationship between blood and urine glucose (e.g. renal threshold varies considerably within and between individuals, where urine glucose excretion is affected by state of hydration etc, see Assessing control in diabetes, p. 67).

Figure 3.6
Simultaneous blood and urinary glucose concentrations.

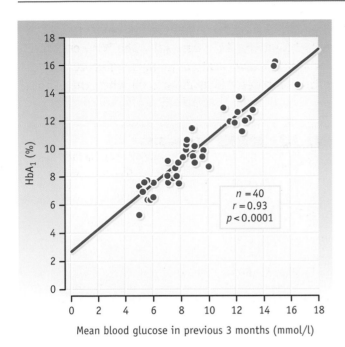

$$n = 40$$
$$r = 0.93$$
$$p < 0.0001$$

At present, it is not possible to diagnose diabetes by measuring glycated haemoglobin (HbA$_{1c}$), the measure of integrated blood glucose control over the preceding few weeks (see Assessing control in diabetes, p. 67). This is because HbA$_{1c}$ is difficult to standardise between laboratories and does not yet have the sensitivity to distinguish IGT from diabetes.

Figure 3.7
HbA$_{1c}$ correlates well with previous mean blood glucose levels but is not yet used to diagnose diabetes.

In 1997, an Expert Committee of the American Diabetes Association proposed modifying the diagnostic criteria for diabetes, by lowering the fasting plasma glucose at which diabetes can be diagnosed to 7.0 mmol/l (because a fasting value of 7.8 mmol/l defines a greater degree of hyperglycaemia than a 2-hour value of 11.1 mmol/l). This simple fasting sample is preferred for diagnosis to the more complex 75 g OGTT. Diabetes can also be diagnosed in those with symptoms and a markedly raised blood glucose concentration. Note the inclusion in the ADA criteria of an 'impaired fasting glucose' category, analogous to impaired glucose tolerance (IGT) but diagnosed by the fasting rather than 2-hour glucose value.

ADA Diagnostic criteria, 1997
1 Symptoms + random plasma glucose ≥11.1 mmol/l (≥200 mg/dl)
2 Fasting plasma glucose ≥7.0 mmol/l (≥126 mg/dl)
3 75g OGTT 2 h plasma glucose ≥11.1 mmol/l (≥200 mg/dl)
• Each method confirmed on a subsequent day by any method
• Impaired fasting glucose (IFG) ≥6.1 and <7.0 mmol/l (≥110 and <126 mg/dl)

Figure 3.8
ADA diagnostic criteria, 1997.

Increased risk of type 2 diabetes

- Obesity, especially truncal
- One or more parents or siblings with type 2 diabetes
- Over 70 years of age
- Certain ethnic groups

Increased risk of type 1 diabetes

- One or more siblings with type 1 diabetes

Causes of secondary and other types of diabetes

- Pregnancy
- Pancreatic disease and alcohol abuse
- Cushing's syndrome and other endocrinopathies
- Potentially diabetogenic drugs

Other risk factors for cardiovascular disease ('syndrome X')

- Hypertension
- Dyslipidaemia

Though early detection of diabetes is clearly desirable, neither the value of systematic screening for diabetes nor the method for doing this have been agreed. It is thought that attention should be focused at first on high-risk individuals who are especially likely to develop diabetes.

Figure 3.9
Some 'high-risk' individuals who should be screened for diabetes.

Chapter 4
Classification of diabetes

Diabetes mellitus

- Insulin-dependent diabetes mellitus (IDDM)
- Non-insulin-dependent diabetes mellitus (NIDDM)
  (a) Non-obese
  (b) Obese
- Malnutrition-related diabetes mellitus
- Other types of diabetes mellitus (associated with specific conditions and syndromes)
- Gestational diabetes mellitus

Impaired glucose tolerance (IGT)

- Non-obese
- Obese
- Associated with certain conditions and syndromes

Figure 4.1
WHO classification of diabetes and impaired glucose tolerance.

The WHO classification of diabetes (1980, revised 1985) included the two common types of diabetes which were identified and classified by a clinical description of the patients, i.e. having either insulin-dependent diabetes mellitus (type 1 diabetes), because they are judged to need insulin to survive, or non-insulin-dependent diabetes mellitus (type 2 diabetes), where insulin deficiency is less severe and insulin replacement is not essential to preserve life. Type 2 diabetes patients may be obese or non-obese. A recent WHO consultation document (1998) proposes a revised classification similar to that of the ADA (see below).

Diabetes due to pancreatic disease

- Chronic or recurrent pancreatitis
- Haemochromatosis

Diabetes due to other endocrine disease

- Cushing's syndrome
- Acromegaly
- Phaeochromocytoma
- Glucagonoma

Diabetes due to drugs and chemicals

- Glucocorticoids and corticotrophin
- Diuretics
- β-blockers

Diabetes due to abnormalities of insulin or its receptor

- Insulinopathies
- Insulin receptor defects
- Circulating antireceptor antibodies

Diabetes associated with genetic syndromes

- DIDMOAD syndrome
- Lipoatrophic diabetes
- Cystic fibrosis

Figure 4.2
Some other types of diabetes.

The classification also includes malnutrition-related diabetes, a rare type of diabetes occurring in the tropics in association with malnutrition. Its aetiology is uncertain and in recent years its status as a separate type of diabetes has been re-evaluated. The ADA has suggested omitting it from the classification. The remaining types of diabetes are 'gestational diabetes', where diabetes occurs for the first time in pregnancy, and other types associated with conditions such as hormone-secreting tumours (e.g. acromegaly, Cushing's syndrome), drugs, pancreatic disease and genetic syndromes.

IDDM (type 1 diabetes)	NIDDM (type 2 diabetes)
Sudden onset	Gradual onset
Severe symptoms, including coma in some patients	May be no symptoms
Recent weight loss	Often no weight loss
Usually lean	Usually obese
Spontaneous ketosis	Not ketotic
Absent C peptide	C peptide detectable
Markers of autoimmunity present (e.g. islet cell antibodies)	No markers of autoimmunity

Other clinical and biochemical features can be used to decide whether the patient has type 1 diabetes or type 2 diabetes.

Figure 4.3
Type 1 or type 2 diabetes?

Impaired glucose tolerance (IGT), not a form of frank diabetes but a lesser degree of glucose intolerance, is defined from the results of an oral glucose tolerance test. IGT has specific clinical implications, being associated with an increased frequency of cardiovascular disease compared to people of normal glucose tolerance, but not associated with an increased frequency of microangiopathy. About 2–5% of people with IGT per year progress to diabetes, but many also revert to normal glucose tolerance on retesting.

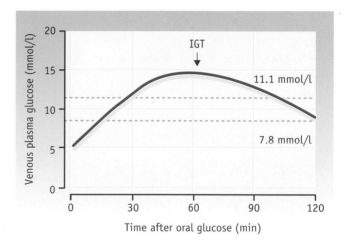

Figure 4.4
Oral glucose tolerance test showing IGT.

For many years, most clinicians have used the terms type 1 and type 2 diabetes synonymously with IDDM and NIDDM respectively. The new classification proposed by the ADA in 1997 abandons the terms IDDM and NIDDM, which may be confusing because they are based on treatment and not aetiology, and retains the terms type 1 and type 2 diabetes. Most cases of type 1 diabetes are due to autoimmune destruction of the islet B cells; type 2 diabetes is caused by insulin resistance with an insulin secretory defect. Malnutrition-related diabetes has been omitted from the ADA classification. IGT is retained with an analogous term 'impaired fasting glucose' (IFG) used for the lesser degree of glucose intolerance when diagnosed by fasting glucose levels. A WHO consultation document (1998) proposes a very similar classification.

ADA Classification of diabetes: 1997

1 Type 1 diabetes (equivalent to IDDM)
   Immune mediated
   Idiopathic

2 Type 2 diabetes (equivalent to NIDDM)
3 Other specific types
4 Gestational diabetes mellitus

Figure 4.5
ADA classification of diabetes, 1997.

Chapter 5
Public health aspects of diabetes

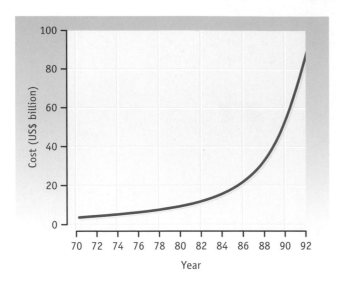

Diabetes is an expensive disease, accounting for at least 5% of health care costs in the UK. The cost of diabetes to the community is increasing, and recent estimates in the USA indicate that the rate of increase is escalating, now accounting for more than US$100 billion per year.

Figure 5.1
The rising costs of diabetes in the USA.

	Type 1 (%)	Type 2 (%)
Cardiovascular disease	15	58
Cerebrovascular disease	3	12
Nephropathy	55	3
Diabetic coma	4	1
Malignancy	0	11
Infections	10	4
Others	13	11

Overall life expectancy in the diabetic patient is reduced by about 25%. The causes of death differ in type 1 and type 2 diabetes. In type 1 diabetes, nephropathy and heart disease are common, whereas in type 2 diabetes most deaths are due to cardiovascular disease, including stroke.

Figure 5.2
Causes of mortality in type 1 and type 2 diabetes.

Diabetes is a rapidly growing problem in the developing world, especially in urban populations of these countries. Practical management is often made difficult by the scarcity of health-care personnel, drugs, monitoring equipment and even food. Premature mortality is much higher in developing countries than in Westernised countries. Potentially avoidable or treatable conditions such as hypoglycaemia, ketoacidosis and infection are common causes of death.

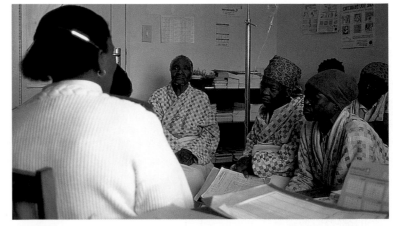

Figure 5.3
A morning education session, led by a nursing sister, at Baragwanath Hospital in Soweto, South Africa. All these patients had been admitted with diabetic emergencies during the preceding 24 hours.

Chapter 6

Normal physiology of insulin secretion and action

HANDBOOK OF DIABETES *2ND EDITION*

Insulin is synthesised in and secreted from the B cells within the islets of Langerhans in the pancreas. The normal pancreas has about 1 million islets. The islets can be easily identified with various histological stains such as haematoxylin and eosin, where the cells react less intensely than the surrounding exocrine pancreatic tissue.

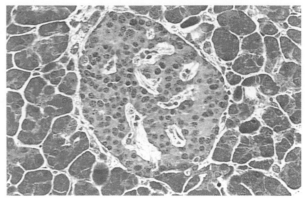

Figure 6.1
A section of normal pancreas stained with haematoxylin and eosin. The islet in the centre is easily identified by its distinct morphology and lighter staining than the surrounding exocrine tissue.

The main cell types of the islet are the B or β cells (producing insulin), the A or α cells (producing glucagon), the D or δ cells (producing somatostatin) and the PP cells (producing pancreatic polypeptide). The different cell types can be identified by immuno-staining techniques. The B cells are the most numerous and are mainly located in the core of the islet, whilst A and D cells are located in the periphery.

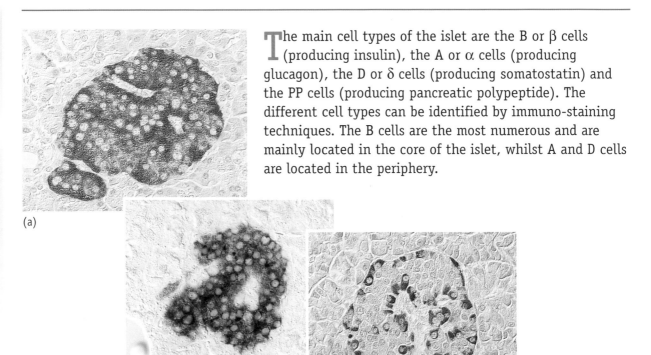

(a)

(b)

(c)

(d)

Figure 6.2
The localisation of pancreatic hormones in human islets.
(a) Insulin immunostained in the majority of cells, forming the core of the islet (peroxidase-antiperoxidase immunostain with haematoxylin counterstain). (b) Insulin mRNA localised by in situ hybridisation with a digoxigenin-labelled sequence of rat insulin cRNA (which crossreacts fully with human insulin mRNA). (c) Peripherally located A cells immunostained with antibodies to pancreatic glucagon using the same method as for (a). (d) Weakly immunoreactive PP cells in the epithelium of a duct in the ventral portion of the pancreatic head. Magnifications approximately × 150.

HANDBOOK OF DIABETES *2ND EDITION*

Islet cells interact with each other through direct contact and through their products, e.g. glucagon stimulates insulin secretion and somatostatin inhibits insulin and glucagon secretion. Islet parasympathetic innervation from the vagus stimulates insulin release, and adrenergic sympathetic nerves inhibit insulin and stimulate glucagon release. There are also nerves originating within the pancreas containing peptides such as vasoactive intestinal peptide (VIP) and neuropeptide Y (NPY) (peptidergic nerves), but their importance in controlling islet cell secretion is unclear.

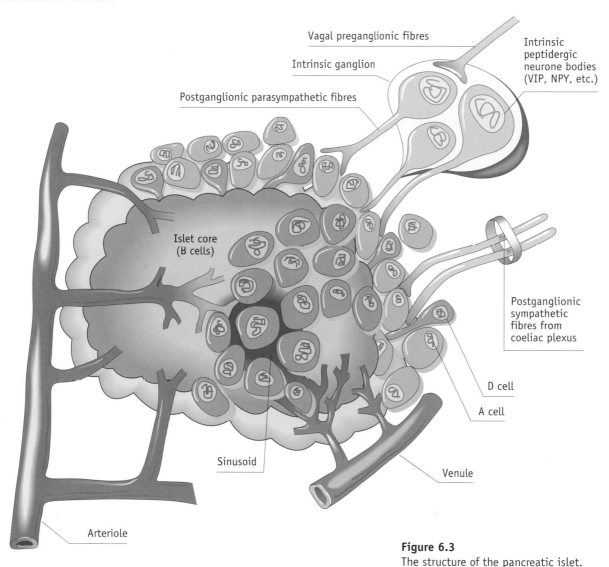

Vagal preganglionic fibres

Intrinsic ganglion

Intrinsic peptidergic neurone bodies (VIP, NPY, etc.)

Postganglionic parasympathetic fibres

Islet core (B cells)

Postganglionic sympathetic fibres from coeliac plexus

D cell

A cell

Sinusoid

Venule

Arteriole

Figure 6.3
The structure of the pancreatic islet.

The insulin molecule consists of two polypeptide chains linked by disulphide bridges, the A chain containing 21 amino acids and the B chain 30 amino acids. Human insulin differs from pig insulin, an animal insulin which has been used extensively for diabetes treatment, at only one amino acid position (B30). Beef insulin—also used therapeutically—differs at three positions (B30, A8 and A10).

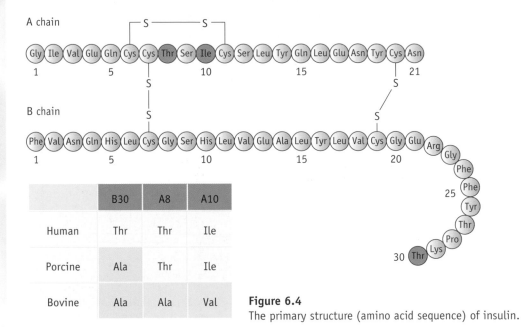

	B30	A8	A10
Human	Thr	Thr	Ile
Porcine	Ala	Thr	Ile
Bovine	Ala	Ala	Val

Figure 6.4
The primary structure (amino acid sequence) of insulin.

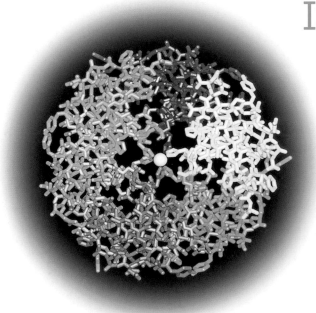

Figure 6.5
The insulin hexamer with each of the six molecules coloured differently.

In dilute solution such as in the bloodstream, insulin exists as the 6000 Da molecular-weight monomer. In concentrated solution and crystals, such as in the insulin secretory granule and in vials of insulin solution supplied by the pharmaceutical companies for insulin injection, six monomers self-associate with two zinc ions to form a hexamer. This is of therapeutic importance because the slow absorption of insulin from subcutaneous tissue is partly due to the time taken for hexameric insulin to disperse and dissociate into the smaller monomeric form (see Management of type 1 diabetes, p. 75).

Insulin is formed in the islet B cells from a single amino acid chain precursor molecule called proinsulin. Synthesis begins with the formation of preproinsulin, which is cleaved by protease activity to proinsulin. The gene for preproinsulin (and therefore 'the gene for insulin') is located on chromosome 11. Proinsulin is packaged into vesicles in the Golgi apparatus of the cell, and in the maturing secretory granules it is converted by enzymes into insulin and connecting peptide (C peptide).

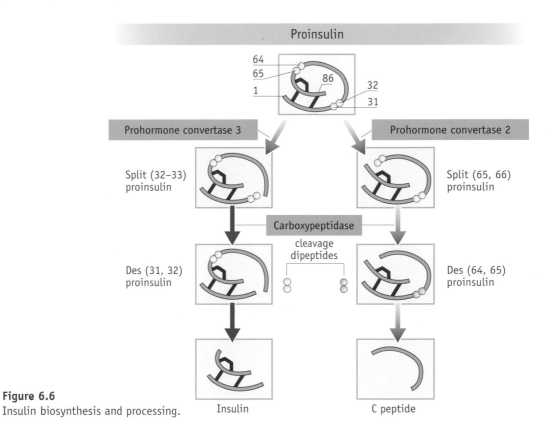

Figure 6.6
Insulin biosynthesis and processing.

Insulin and C peptide are released (exocytosis) from the B cell when the granules are transported ('translocated') to the cell surface and the granule membrane fuses with the plasma membrane of the B cell. Microtubules and microfilaments are involved in the translocation process.

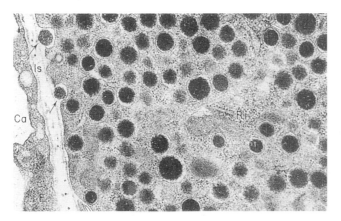

Figure 6.7
Electron micrograph of insulin storage granules in a pancreatic B cell. The arrows show granules undergoing exocytosis.

Under some circumstances, such as in type 2 diabetes and insulinoma, the normal packaging and conversion of proinsulin in granules (regulated pathway) is bypassed and an alternative, constitutive pathway operates where more of the proinsulin is secreted as vesicles directly originating from the Golgi apparatus. Therefore, more intact proinsulin and incompletely processed products ('split proinsulins') are released.

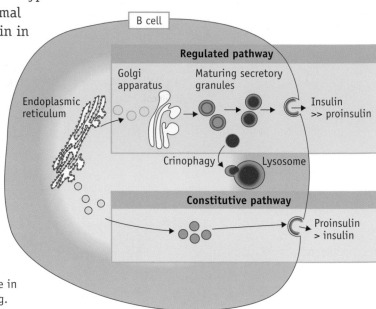

Figure 6.8
The regulated (normal) and constitutive (active in type 2 diabetes) pathways of insulin processing.

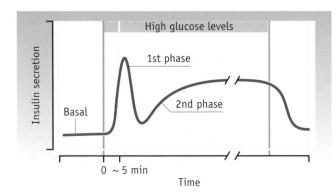

Glucose is the main stimulator of insulin release from the B cell, which occurs in a characteristic biphasic pattern—an acute, first phase lasting only a few minutes, followed by a sustained second phase.

Figure 6.9
The biphasic glucose-stimulated release of insulin from the B cell.

The mechanism by which glucose stimulates insulin release probably involves initial entry into the B cell via a glucose transporter (GLUT 2) which is closely associated with the enzyme glucokinase. This phosphorylates glucose and is the essential glucose sensor of the B cell. In order for insulin release to occur, glucose must be metabolised within the B cell, via glycolysis, to produce ATP. This closes ATP-sensitive potassium channels, causing depolarisation, which then leads to an influx of calcium ions, triggering granule translocation and exocytosis. Note that the class of oral hypoglycaemic drugs which stimulate insulin secretion, sulphonylureas, also act in a similar way by binding to a receptor and closing potassium channels (see Management of type 2 diabetes, p. 87).

Figure 6.10
Possible mechanism by which glucose stimulates insulin secretion.

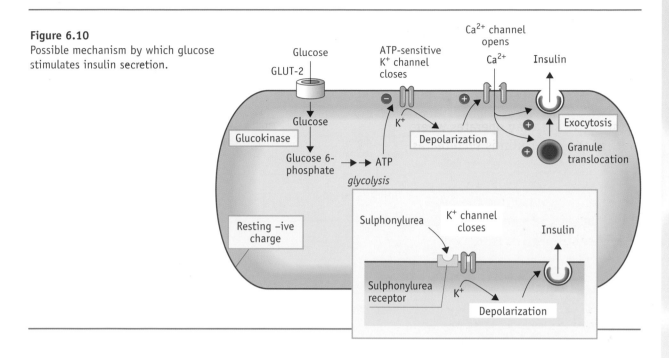

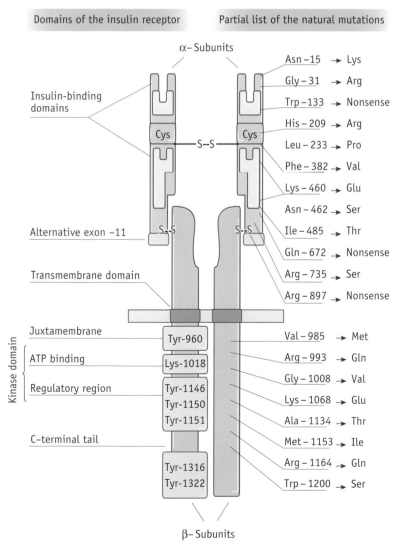

Insulin exerts its biological effects by binding to a receptor on the target cell surface. The insulin receptor is a glycoprotein consisting of two extracellular α subunits and two β subunits, which are partly intracellular. The receptor has tyrosine kinase enzymatic activity (residing in the β subunit) which is stimulated when insulin binds to the receptor. This activity then phosphorylates tyrosine amino-acid residues on various intracellular proteins, as well as the receptor itself (autophosphorylation). Tyrosine kinase activity is essential for insulin action.

Figure 6.11
The insulin receptor and its structural domains. Many mutations have been discovered in the insulin; some are shown here.

Many of the postreceptor signalling mechanisms for insulin are unknown, but a major cytoplasmic substrate for the enzymatic activity of the receptor is a 131-kDa protein called insulin-receptor substrate 1 (IRS-1). IRS-1 has 22 potential tyrosine phosphorylation sites; rapid phosphorylation leads to non-covalent binding between the phosphorylated sites of IRS-1 and specific domains (SH2 domains) on target proteins in the cell such as PI_3-kinase (phosphatidylinositol 3-kinase) and GRB2. The mechanisms by which the binding of IRS-1 to SH2 proteins lead to the various actions of insulin is incompletely understood.

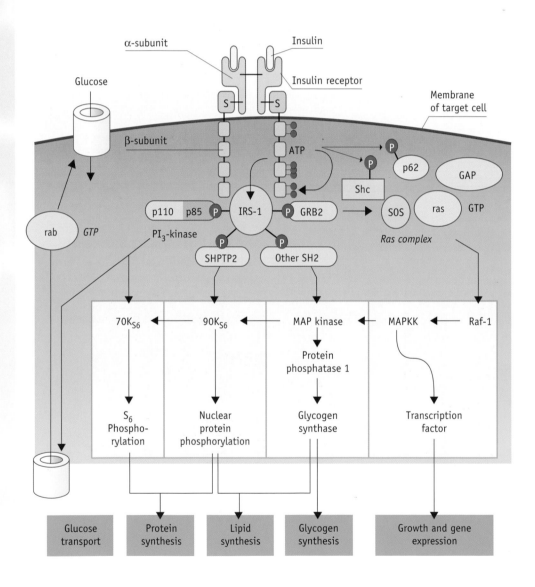

Figure 6.12
Insulin signalling pathways.

HANDBOOK OF DIABETES 2ND EDITION

After binding of insulin to its receptor, the insulin-receptor complex is internalised by the surrounding membrane invaginating to form an 'endosome'. The receptors are recycled to the cell surface, but insulin is degraded in lysosomes. The protein clathrin plays a key role in this process. Elevated insulin levels, as in obesity and type 2 diabetes, lead to 'down-regulation' of the receptor, where internalisation results in decreased numbers at the cell surface.

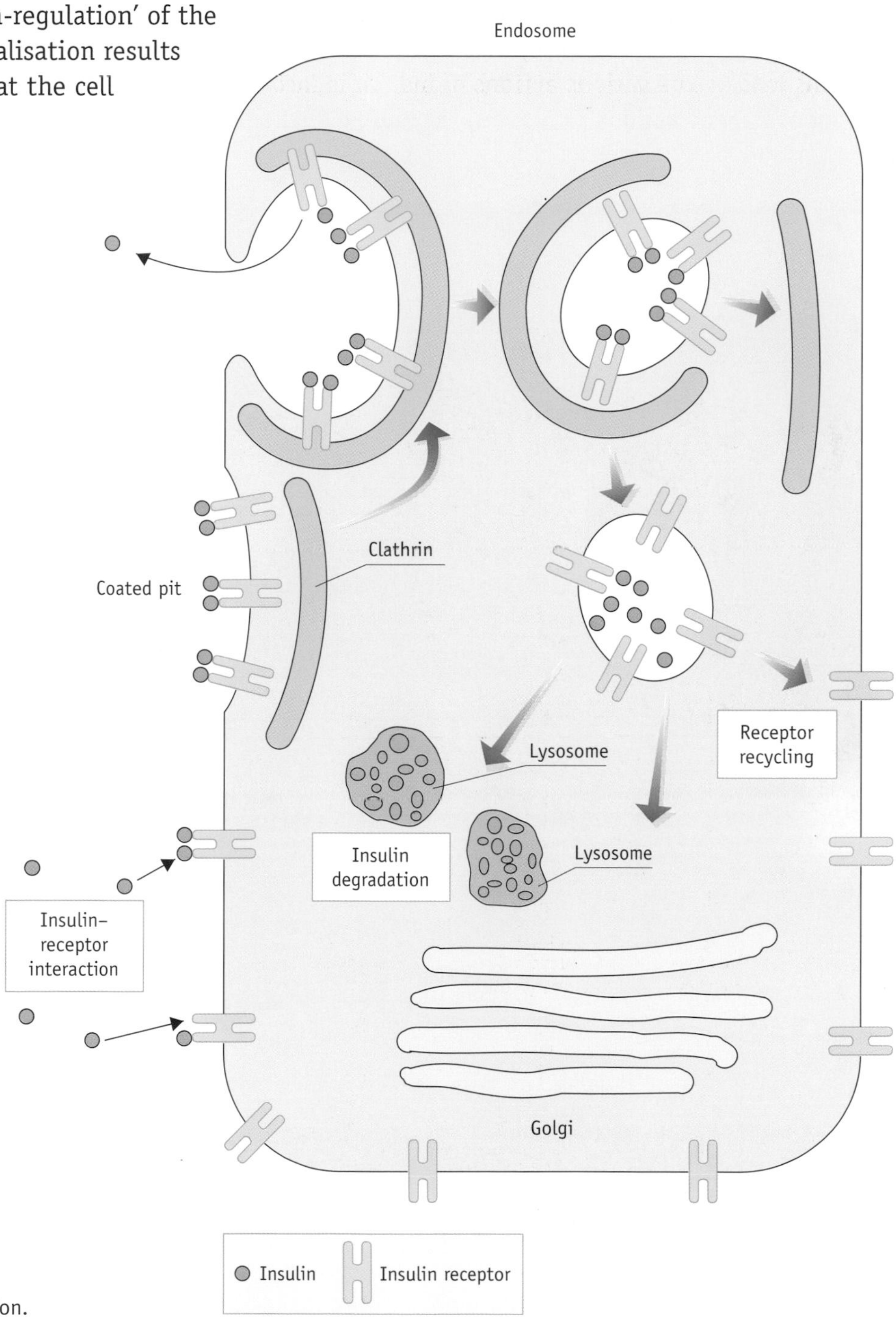

Figure 6.13
Insulin receptor internalisation.

Glucose is carried into cells across the cell membrane by a family of specialised transporter proteins called glucose transporters (GLUTs):

- GLUT-1 is involved in basal and non-insulin-mediated glucose uptake in many cells;
- GLUT-2 is important in the islet B cell, where it is a prerequisite with glucokinase, for glucose sensing;
- GLUT-3 is involved in non-insulin-mediated uptake of glucose in the brain;
- GLUT-4 is responsible for insulin-stimulated glucose uptake—one of the classical hypoglycaemic actions of insulin—in muscle, and adipose tissue.

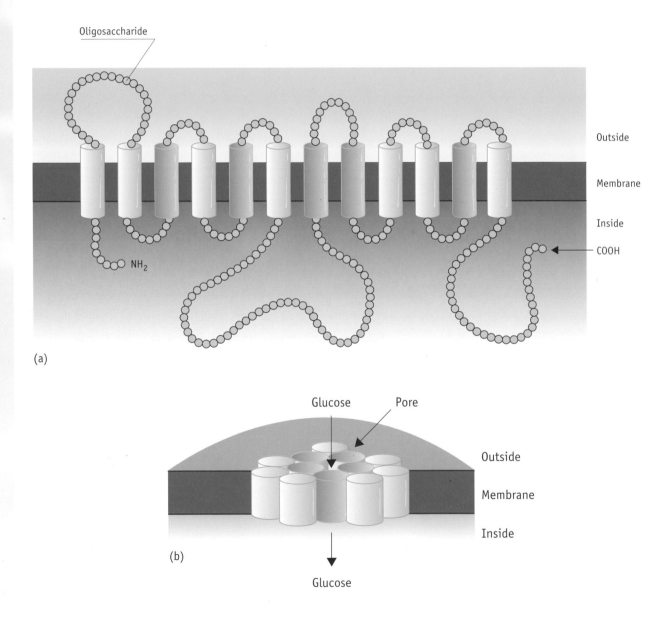

(a)

(b)

Figure 6.14
(a) The structure of a typical GLUT. (b) The intramembrane domains may pack together to form a central hydrophilic channel through which glucose passes.

HANDBOOK OF DIABETES 2ND EDITION

GLUT-4 is normally located in vesicles in the cytoplasm. Insulin recruits the vesicles and causes them to be translocated to the cell surface where GLUT-4 functions as a pore for glucose entry. Exercise has a similar effect on GLUT-4.

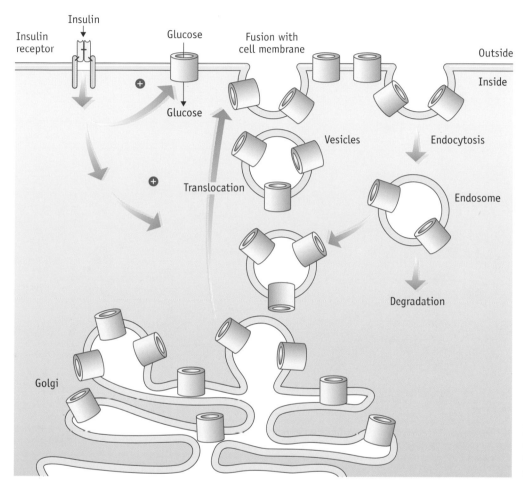

Figure 6.15
Insulin regulation of glucose transport into cells via GLUT-4.

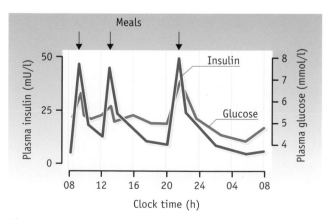

Figure 6.16
Blood profiles of glucose and insulin in non-diabetic individuals.

In normal subjects, blood glucose levels are maintained within relatively narrow limits at around 5 mmol/l (90 mg/dl) by the balance between glucose entry into the bloodstream from the liver and from intestinal absorption after meals, and glucose uptake into the peripheral tissues such as muscle. Insulin is secreted as a low, basal level between meals and at an increased, stimulated level at mealtimes.

Figure 6.17

Overview of carbohydrate metabolism. Cats, catecholamines; cort, cortisol; glcg, glucagon; ins, insulin; NIMGU, non-insulin-mediated glucose uptake.

The brain consumes about 80% of the glucose utilised at rest in the fasting state, but glucose uptake into the brain is not regulated by insulin. Glucose is the main fuel for the brain, so that the brain depends critically on the maintenance of normal blood glucose levels.

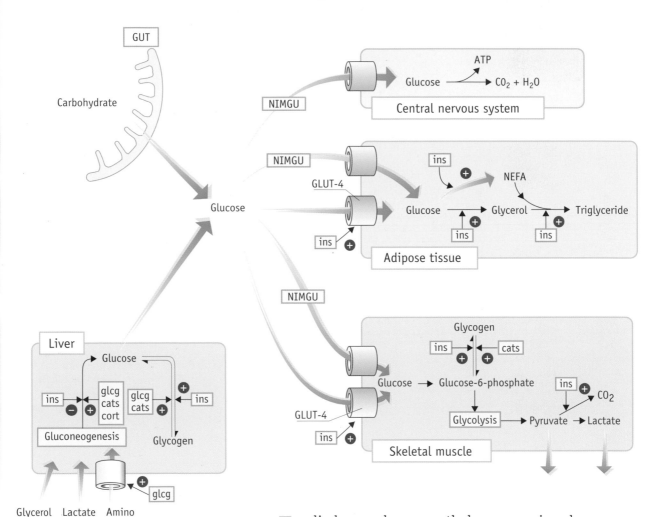

Insulin lowers glucose partly by suppressing glucose output from the liver (i.e. by inhibiting glycogen breakdown—glycogenolysis—and by inhibiting gluconeogenesis, the formation of 'new' glucose from sources such as glycerol, lactate and amino acids like alanine). Relatively low amounts of insulin are needed to suppress hepatic glucose output, such as occurs with basal insulin secretion. With higher concentrations of insulin, such as occur after meals, glucose uptake into the periphery (adipose tissue, muscle) is stimulated, mediated by GLUT-4.

Chapter 7

Epidemiology
and aetiology
of type 1 diabetes

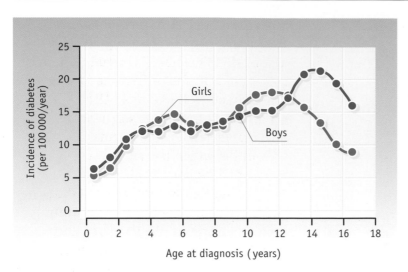

Figure 7.1
Age-specific incidence of type 1 diabetes showing peaks at pre-school age and later around puberty.

Although type 1 diabetes can occur at all ages, it predominantly arises in children and young adults, with a peak incidence before school age and again at around puberty. The age at onset is similar for both girls and boys, though the pubertal peak possibly occurs earlier in girls.

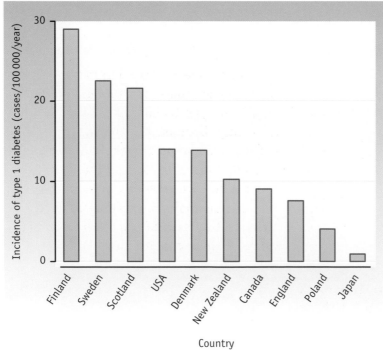

Figure 7.2
Geographical variation in the incidence of type 1 diabetes.

There is a marked geographical variation in the incidence of type 1 diabetes, with Northern European countries like Finland and Sweden showing very high frequencies (up to 30–35 cases per year per 100 000 of the population) and Oriental countries such as Japan, China and Korea showing a low incidence (about 0.5–2.0 cases per year per 100 000 population). This difference in frequency suggests that environmental or ethnic factors may influence the onset of the disease.

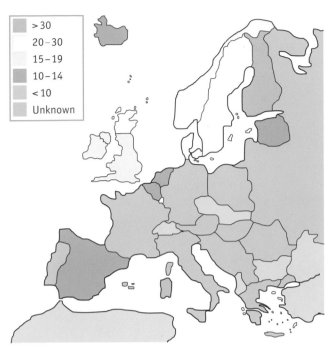

Figure 7.3
Incidence rates (cases per 100 000/year) of type 1 diabetes (onset 0–14 years) in Europe. Note the high incidence in Nordic countries, Scotland and Sardinia.

The geographical variation within Europe has recently been highlighted in the EURODIAB epidemiological study. There is more than a 10-fold difference in incidence from Finland to Macedonia. Although there is a tendency towards a North–South gradient, remarkable 'hot spots' occur, such as Sardinia, which has an incidence several-fold higher than those of surrounding Mediterranean populations. The different incidences in genetically similar countries such as Finland and Estonia or Norway and Iceland suggests environmental influences may predominate over genetic susceptibility in causing or triggering the disease.

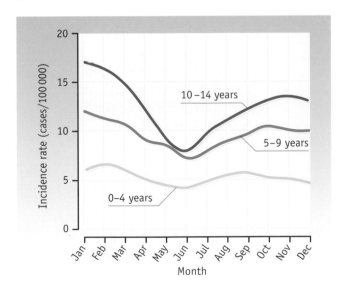

Figure 7.4
Incidence rates of type 1 diabetes according to months of clinical onset and age groups in both boys and girls.

Further evidence for environmental influences comes from studies which show that type 1 diabetes is more commonly diagnosed in the winter months. This might represent increasing demands for insulin during the winter (glucose tolerance deteriorates in the winter in normal subjects) or seasonal exposure to precipitating environmental agents such as viruses.

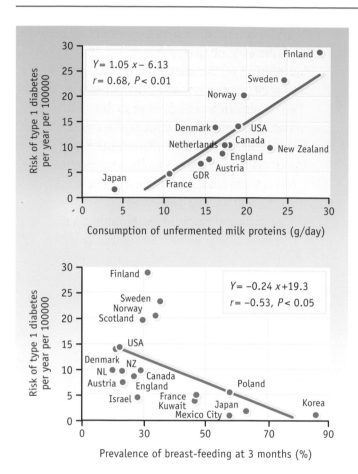

In addition to viruses, a possible environmental determinant of type 1 diabetes is food. For example, exposure in women to nitrosamines in smoked meat eaten at the time of conception increases the occurrence of type 1 diabetes in their children. An association between low frequency of breast feeding and high risk of type 1 diabetes has not been confirmed in all studies, but it may point to a causal role for cow's milk protein in some cases. It is postulated that antibodies to bovine serum albumin (a major protein of cow's milk) might cross react with specific islet B-cell components.

Figure 7.5
The relationship between risk of type 1 diabetes and the consumption of milk protein (top) and the prevalence of breast-feeding (bottom) in different countries.

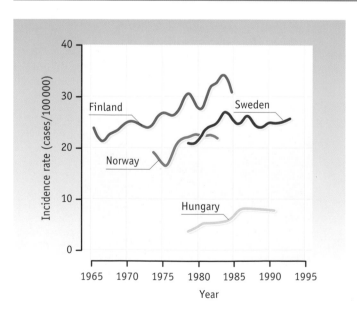

The incidence of type 1 diabetes is increasing in several countries where frequencies have been studied over a number of years (e.g. Finland, Sweden, Norway, Hungary, Denmark, the Netherlands, Poland, Sardinia, the UK and some populations in the USA).

Figure 7.6
Secular trends in standardised incidence of type 1 diabetes in children aged 0–14 years in various European populations.

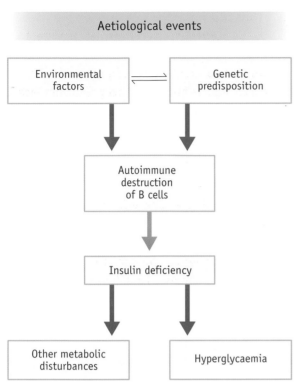

Aetiological events

Environmental factors

Genetic predisposition

Autoimmune destruction of B cells

Insulin deficiency

Other metabolic disturbances

Hyperglycaemia

The commonest cause of type 1 diabetes (over 90% of cases) is autoimmune destruction of the islet B cells. The exact aetiology is complex and still imperfectly understood. However, it is probable that environmental factors trigger the onset of diabetes in individuals with an inherited predisposition. Unless insulin replacement is given, severe insulin deficiency results in hyperglycaemia and ketoacidosis, the biochemical hallmark of type 1 diabetes.

Figure 7.7
Aetiology of type 1 diabetes.

Evidence for autoimmunity includes the presence of a chronic inflammatory mononuclear cell infiltrate ('insulitis') associated with the residual B cells in the islets of recently diagnosed type 1 patients. Insulin-secreting B cells are almost totally absent from islets in established type 1 diabetic subjects.

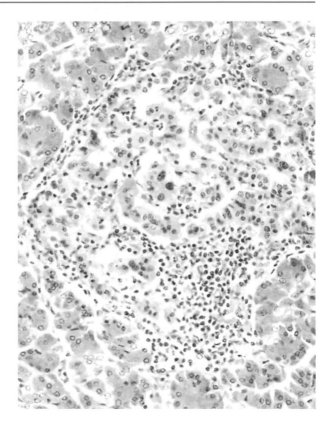

Figure 7.8
Insulitis. Chronic inflammatory cells in islet. Haematoxylin and eosin stain ×300.

HANDBOOK OF DIABETES *2ND EDITION*

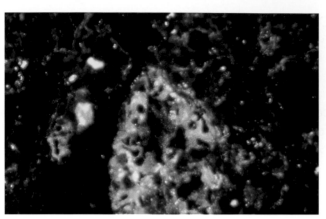

Figure 7.9
ICA demonstrated by indirect immunofluorescence in a frozen section of human pancreas.

Other markers of autoimmunity are islet cell antibodies (ICA, directed at the cytoplasm of all cell types in the islet) and islet cell surface antibodies (more B-cell specific) which are present in the circulation of most newly diagnosed type 1 diabetic subjects. Antibody levels decline with increasing duration of the disease.

There are likely to be several autoantigens reacting with these antibodies, including glutamic acid decarboxylase (GAD). Antibodies to an isoform of this enzyme, GAD65, are present in up to 90% of recent-onset type 1 patients. Insulin autoantibodies are also present in many recent-onset patients. These markers have varying diagnostic and predictive value in type 1 diabetes.

Antibody	Abbreviation	Diagnostic		Predictive value	
		Sensitivity	Specificity	First-degree relatives	General population
Islet-cell antibodies	ICA	80–90%	96–99%	20–50%	20–30%
Islet-cell surface antibodies	ICSA	30–60%	95%	ND	ND
Cytotoxic islet-cell antibodies	C'AMC	40–60%	95%	ND	ND
Insulin autoantibodies	IAA	40–70%	99%	<50%	ND
Glutamate decarboxylase (GAD65)	GAD65AB	70–90%	99%	>50%	ND

Figure 7.10
Various ICA as markers for the development of type 1 diabetes. ND, not determined.

Addison's disease
Graves' disease
Hypothyroidism
Hypogonadism
Pernicious anaemia
Vitiligo

Figure 7.11
Autoimmune disorders associated with type 1 diabetes (autoimmune polyendocrine syndrome).

Type 1 diabetes may accompany other diseases of autoimmune origin such as hypothyroidism, pernicious anaemia and Addison's disease.

Inherited susceptibility to type 1 diabetes depends on several genes at different loci. The strongest linkage is with the human leukocyte antigen (HLA) genes lying within the MHC (major histocompatibility complex) region on the short arm of chromosome 6 (now called 'type 1 diabetes1' locus). HLA antigens are cell surface glycoproteins that shown extreme variability due to polymorphisms in the genes that code for them. Over 95% of Caucasian type 1 diabetic subjects carry HLA-DR3 and/or DR4 (class II antigens) compared to 50% in non-diabetic controls. HLA class II antigens play a key role in presenting foreign- and self-antigens to T lymphocytes and therefore in initiating the autoimmune response.

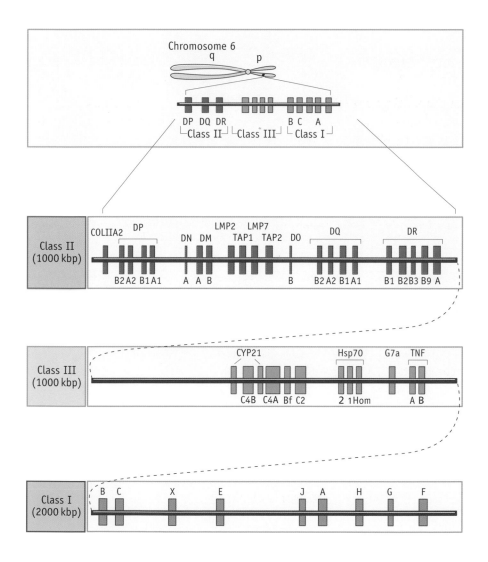

Figure 7.12
A simplified map of the MHC region on the short arm of the chromosome, showing the major genes of classes II, III and I.

HANDBOOK OF DIABETES *2ND EDITION*

These associations can be explained by polymorphisms in the DQB1 gene that result in amino acid substitutions in the class II antigens and may affect the ability to accept and present autoantigens derived from the B cell.

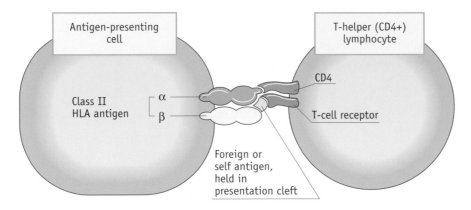

Figure 7.13
Antigen, associated with class II HLA antigen, is presented to T cells.

The region of the insulin gene on chromosome 11 (now called 'type 1 diabetes2') is also linked with type 1 diabetes, possibly because insulin production affects B-cell activity and expression of other autoantigens. Several other loci show weaker linkages with human type 1 diabetes and their nature and importance are being investigated.

Designation	Nature	Chromosome
IDDM1*	MHC	6
IDDM2	Insulin	11
Weaker susceptibility loci:		
IDDM3	?	15
IDDM4	?	11
IDDM5	?	6

Figure 7.14
Susceptibility loci for type 1 diabetes. *Also known as type 1 diabetes1, 2 etc.

The most likely environment agents involved in the aetiology of type 1 diabetes are viruses and dietary components. Viruses may target the islet B cells and destroy them directly or may trigger an autoimmune reaction. This may be because a viral antigen crossreacts with a B-cell antigen, because B-cell antigens are altered and made 'foreign' or because viruses induce aberrant HLA class II antigen on islet B cells, thereby presenting their own surface antigens to T lymphocytes. Islet B-cell damage may be due to cytotoxic T lymphocytes, NK (natural killer) cells, cytokines or autoantibodies.

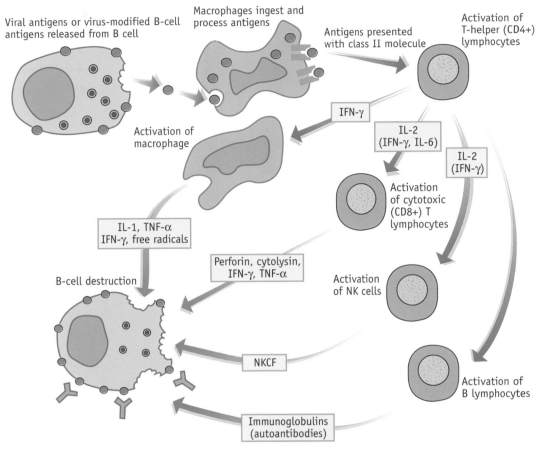

Figure 7.15
Hypothetical scheme showing ways in which viruses could initiate an autoimmune attack on the B cells by inducing them to express autoantigens. Some viruses (e.g. retroviruses) may induce B cells to express viral (foreign) antigens, or render an endogenous B-cell antigen immunogenic. Viral antigens released from the B cells during normal B-cell turnover might be processed by macrophages and presented to T-helper lymphocytes (CD4+), in association with HLA class II antigens.

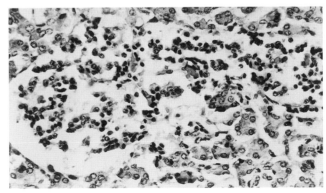

Figure 7.16
Histological section of pancreas from a 10-year-old boy infected with Coxsackie B virus who died soon after developing acute type 1 diabetes, demonstrating extensive insulitis and severe destruction of islet architecture (×160).

Most viruses have been implicated in human diabetes by temporal and geographical associations between type 1 diabetes and a viral infection. For example, mumps occasionally precedes type 1 diabetes, and intrauterine rubella infection induces diabetes in up to 20% of cases. Many people with recent-onset type 1 diabetes have serological or clinical evidence of Coxsackie B virus infection, particularly the B4 serotype. Marked islet B-cell damage has been detected in children who have died from Coxsackie B virus infection.

The notion that there may be environmental B-cell toxins is supported by the existence of chemicals which are known to cause an insulin-dependent type of diabetes in animals. Examples are alloxan and streptozotocin (STZ), both of which damage the B cell at several sites, including membrane disruption, enzyme interaction (e.g. glucokinase) and DNA fragmentation. The rat poison, vacor, causes type 1 diabetes in humans, possibly because it has a similar action to streptozotocin.

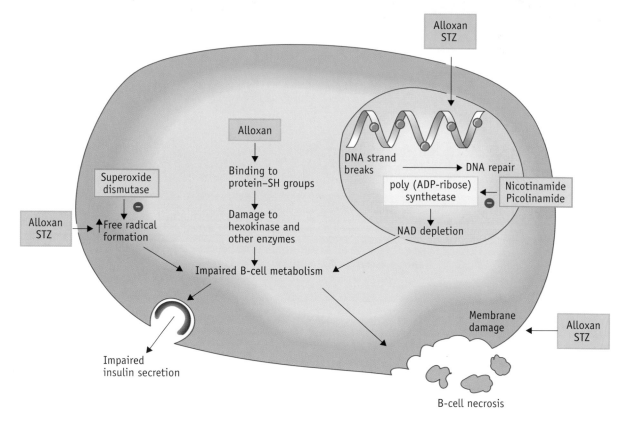

Figure 7.17
Suggested mechanisms of alloxan and streptozotocin toxicity on the B cell. Inhibitors of poly(ADP-ribose) synthetase such as nicotinamide and superoxide dismutase, a free-radical scavenger, can protect against the diabetogenic effects of these agents.

Chapter 8

Epidemiology and aetiology of type 2 diabetes

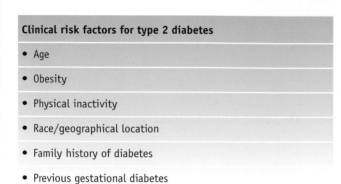

Clinical risk factors for type 2 diabetes
• Age
• Obesity
• Physical inactivity
• Race/geographical location
• Family history of diabetes
• Previous gestational diabetes

Figure 8.1
Clinical risk factors for type 2 diabetes.

Type 2 (non-insulin-dependent) diabetes is the commonest type of diabetes. Various clinical risk factors which are associated with the disease, such as obesity, increasing age, family history of diabetes and ethnic and geographical variations in its frequency, give clues to the aetiology and pathophysiology of type 2 diabetes.

The prevalence of both diabetes and impaired glucose tolerance (IGT) increase with age; each affect about 10–20% of subjects over the age of 65 years in many Western countries. Most subjects are diagnosed after the age of 40 years, the peak age of onset being about 60 years.

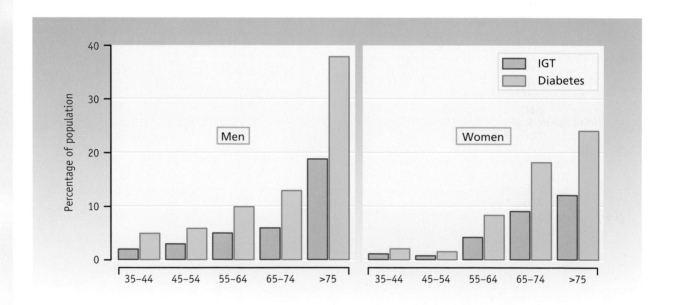

Figure 8.2
Prevalences of IGT and diabetes according to age, in Busselton, Western Australia.

HANDBOOK OF DIABETES *2ND EDITION*

There is a large variation in the frequency of type 2 diabetes in different countries. The highest rates are found in some native American tribes, notably the Pima Indians of Arizona (>50%), and in the South Pacific island of Nauru. These people once had a traditional agricultural lifestyle but have become Westernised relatively rapidly in the last few decades, and are now overweight and inactive. Low prevalence (<1%) is found in poorly developed rural communities such as in parts of Chile and China. In most populations, there are about equal numbers of known and previously undetected cases.

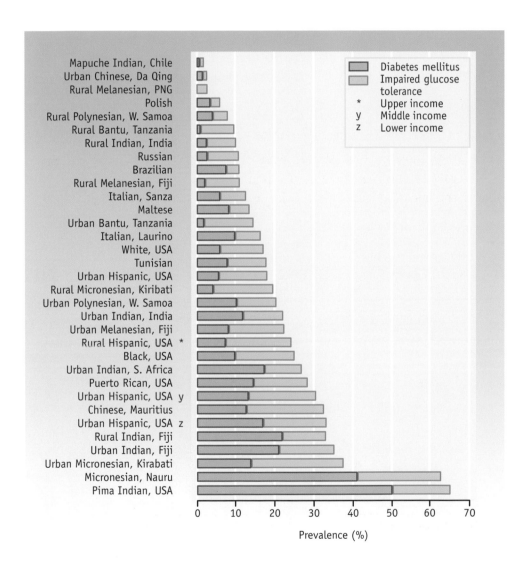

Figure 8.3
Prevalence of diabetes and IGT in selected populations in the age range of 30–64 years.

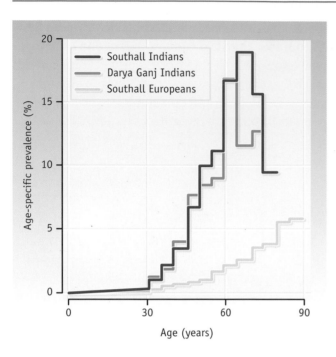

A good example of ethnic effects is seen in the different frequencies of type 2 diabetes amongst the multi-ethnic population in the UK. Considerable migration to Britain occurred in the 1950s and 1960s from the Indian subcontinent and the Caribbean. The frequency of diabetes in Asians is over four times as high as in the local Caucasian population (e.g. the survey in Southall, West London). A similar frequency is found in an affluent suburb (Darya Ganj) of Delhi, India. African-Caribbean people in the UK also have a very high frequency of type 2 diabetes. In the USA there are high rates in black African-Americans and in migrant Hispanic groups (Mexicans and Puerto Ricans).

Figure 8.4
Age-specific prevalence of known diabetes in UK Southall Indians, white Europeans in Southall, Darya Ganj Indians in Delhi, India.

The important role of obesity in type 2 diabetes is shown by the correlation between the degree of fatness in different countries and the frequency of diabetes.

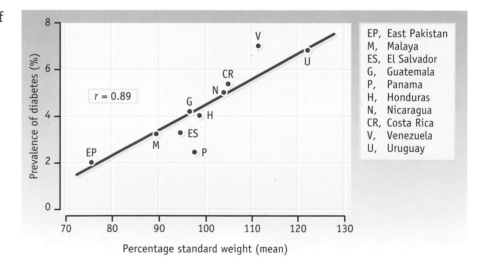

Figure 8.5
Relationship of average fatness and prevalence of diabetes in subjects over 29 years of age in 10 countries.

Aabout 80% of type 2 diabetic patients are obese. The risk of developing diabetes increases progressively in both men and women with the degree of overweight, at least partly due to the decrease in insulin sensitivity as weight increases.

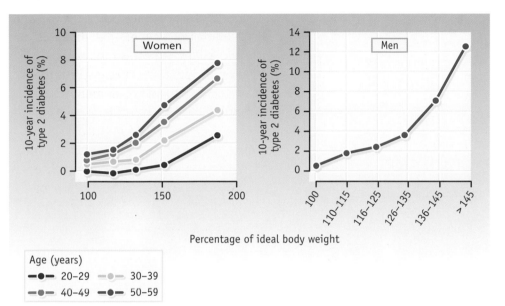

Figure 8.6
Relationship between obesity (expressed as a percentage of ideal body weight) and the 10-year incidence of type 2 diabetes in women and men in the age range of 50–59 years.

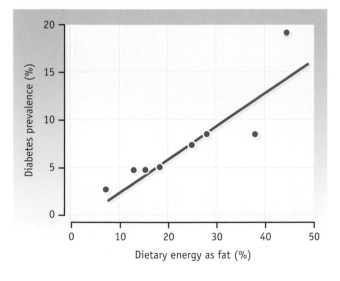

Obesity is related to the amount of fat in the diet, and the prevalence of type 2 diabetes is generally highest in countries with a fat-rich diet. Type of dietary fat is important as Eskimos and Japanese, who have a high-fat but fish-based diet, have a low frequency of diabetes.

Figure 8.7
Prevalence of diabetes in different populations is associated with the fat content of the diet (exceptions being the Eskimos and Japanese).

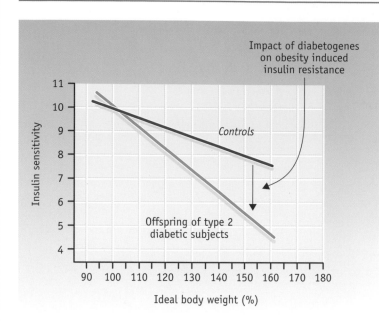

Two important factors which increase the impact of obesity are the genetic background of the patient and the distribution of the obesity. Subjects with a strong family history of diabetes (both parents with type 2 diabetes) become more insulin resistant as weight increases than subjects with no family history of type 2 diabetes.

Figure 8.8
Interaction between obesity and genetic predisposition to type 2 diabetes on insulin sensitivity.

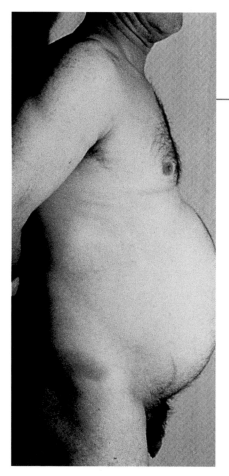

The greatest risk of diabetes is associated with central or truncal obesity where fat is deposited subcutaneously and at intra-abdominal sites. This type of obesity is more typical of men and is therefore known as 'android'. In clinical practice, central obesity can be assessed by the weight : hip ratio of body circumference, but simple measurements of waist circumference are also useful.

Figure 8.9
Central or truncal obesity in a man.

Visceral fat (accumulated in central obesity) is more metabolically active than peripheral fat and releases large quantities of non-esterified fatty acids (NEFA). NEFA have several metabolic actions that can cause insulin resistance, such as stimulating gluconeogenesis in the liver and inhibiting glucose uptake in muscle.

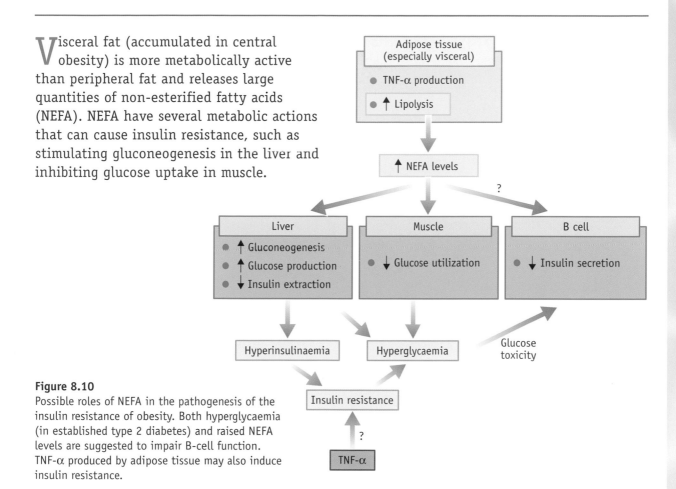

Figure 8.10
Possible roles of NEFA in the pathogenesis of the insulin resistance of obesity. Both hyperglycaemia (in established type 2 diabetes) and raised NEFA levels are suggested to impair B-cell function. TNF-α produced by adipose tissue may also induce insulin resistance.

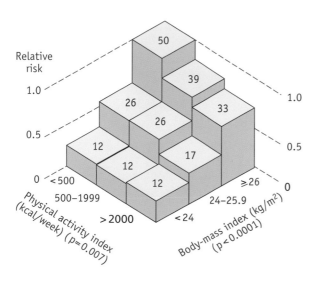

Low levels of physical exercise also predict the development of type 2 diabetes, possibly due to the effect of exercise in increasing insulin sensitivity and preventing obesity.

Figure 8.11
Age-adjusted risk of type 2 diabetes among 5990 men. The figure shows data for the physical activity index in relation to BMI. Each block represents the relative risk of type 2 diabetes per 10 000 man-years of follow-up, with the risk for the tallest block set at 1.0. The numbers on the blocks are incidence rates of type 2 diabetes per 10 000 man-years.

HANDBOOK OF DIABETES *2ND EDITION*

Evidence for a genetic basis to type 2 diabetes includes family clustering of insulin sensitivity, for example in the Pima Indians with diabetes. Some families have members who all have a low insulin sensitivity and some have members where all have a high sensitivity.

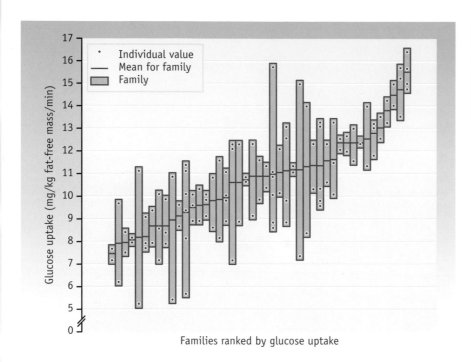

Families ranked by glucose uptake

Figure 8.12
Dispersion of whole-body glucose uptake under glucose clamp conditions (an index of insulin sensitivity), within and between families of Pima Indians.

Twin studies provide further evidence for genetic factors in type 2 diabetes, though the interpretation is controversial. Early reports showed that there was a 60–100% concordance for the disease in identical (monozygotic) twins, but later studies with random recruitment show rates of about 33% in monozygotic twins. Part of the explanation for the concordance in twins may be non-genetic, in that these twins usually share a single placenta and are influenced by the same intrauterine metabolic environment (see 'thrifty phenotype' hypothesis).

Figure 8.13
Twins provide evidence for a genetic basis to type 2 diabetes.

HANDBOOK OF DIABETES *2ND EDITION*

There are many potential 'diabetogenes', i.e. candidate genes involved in controlling insulin secretion and action which may play a role in type 2 diabetes. In the common type of non-insulin-dependent diabetes, no convincingly important abnormalities have been found yet amongst the many genes investigated.

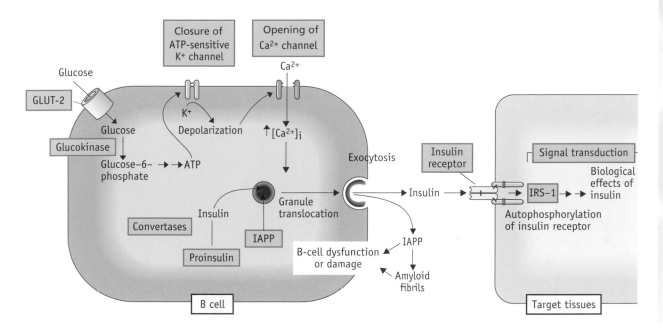

Figure 8.14
Key steps in insulin secretion and insulin action, showing some possible candidate genes for type 2 diabetes (highlighted in green).

One rare type of diabetes (up to 1% of diabetes in white populations) where definite gene defects have been identified is maturity-onset diabetes of the young (MODY). This is a non-insulin-dependent diabetes with onset before the age of 25 years, inherited in an autosomal dominant manner. It is primarily due to an islet B-cell defect and there is no significant insulin resistance. Mutations in glucokinase (responsible for glucose sensing) and in hepatic nuclear factors 1α and 4α (transcription factors regulating gene expression) have been detected in various affected families.

	HNF-4a (MODY1)	Glucokinase (MODY2)	HNF-1a (MODY3)
Frequency	5%	10%	65%
Chromosome location	20q	7q	12q

Figure 8.15
Common mutations causing MODY, and their designations.

The influence of intrauterine and neonatal nutrition on the later development of type 2 diabetes has been emphasised recently in the 'thrifty phenotype' hypothesis. Original observations centred on a study of birth weights in a cohort of men born in 1920–30 in Hertfordshire, UK. Those with the lowest birth weight had the highest frequency of type 2 diabetes in adult life. Hales and Barker thus proposed that fetal and early childhood malnutrition 'programmes' metabolism by impairing B-cell development and inducing insulin resistance. If nutrition is abundant in adult life, leading to obesity, diabetes and IGT result. Further studies have shown that coronary heart disease, hypertension and dyslipidaemia (syndrome X) are also associated with low birth weight.

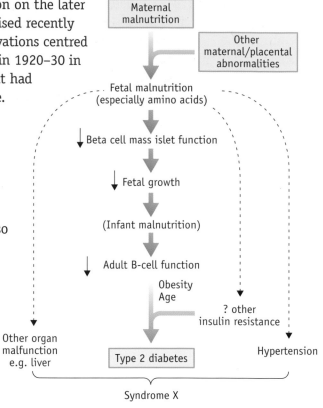

Figure 8.16
The 'thrifty phenotype' hypothesis.

The two main pathophysiological defects in type 2 diabetes are impaired insulin secretion and insulin resistance. The main B-cell abnormalities include a markedly reduced first-phase insulin secretion in response to glucose, and in established diabetes an attenuated second phase. Insulin pulsatility is also abnormal in type 2 diabetes, thereby reducing tissue insulin sensitivity, and the processing of proinsulin to insulin is impaired leading to oversecretion of proinsulin and its 'split' products.

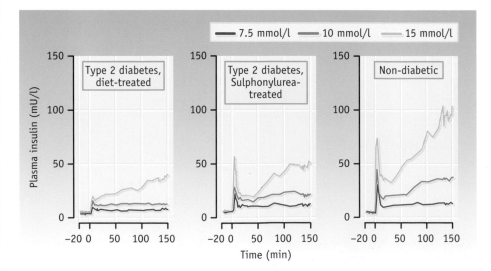

Figure 8.17
Insulin secretory profiles in non-diabetic and subjects with type 2 diabetes during studies in which the plasma glucose concentration was maintained at 7.5, 10 or 15 mmol/l. First-phase responses are virtually absent in patients with type 2 diabetes who were treated with diet alone, and are substantially restored by sulphonylurea treatment in type 2 diabetes.

HANDBOOK OF DIABETES 2ND EDITION

Impaired meal-related insulin secretion in type 2 diabetes leads to exaggerated and prolonged postprandial hyperglycaemia, which is an important contributor to the overall loss of glycaemic control. The realisation of the importance of postprandial glucose regulation and the evidence in some trials that postprandial, but not fasting hyperglycaemia is a risk factor for cardiovascular disease in type 2 diabetes has encouraged the development of treatments specifically aimed at reduction of postprandial blood glucose levels (see Management of type 2 diabetes, p. 87).

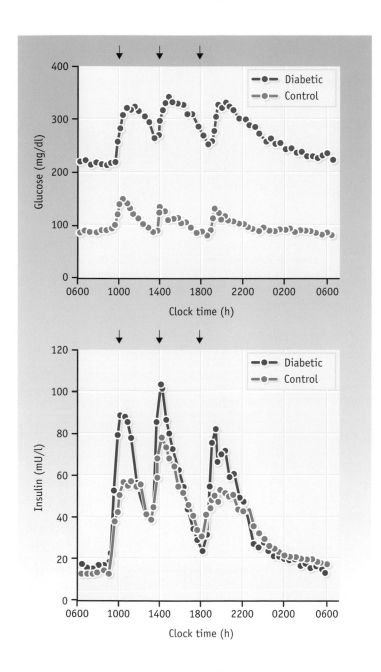

Figure 8.18
Concentrations of glucose and insulin in diabetic and control subjects.
Times at which meals were served are indicated by arrows.

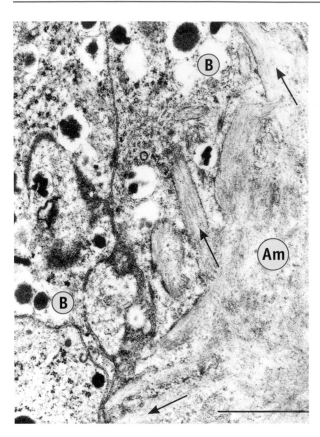

The main histological abnormality in the islets of type 2 diabetic patients is the presence of amyloid, insoluble fibrils formed outside of cells derived from the peptide IAPP (islet amyloid polypeptide or amylin). IAPP is produced in the islet B cells and co-secreted with insulin. At high concentrations, IAPP inhibits insulin secretion, but it is unclear what part islet amyloid or IAPP play in the pathology of type 2 diabetes.

Figure 8.19
Electron micrograph appearances of islet amyloid deposits in type 2 diabetes; amyloid (Am) fibrils closely surround the B cells (B) and deeply invaginate the distorted cell membrane. Scale bar, 1 μm.

Insulin resistance can be demonstrated in type 2 diabetes by several methods, including the euglycaemic glucose clamp, when insulin is infused intravenously and the amount of intravenous glucose to achieve constant glucose concentrations is measured. Although insulin sensitivity is low in those with type 2 diabetes, resistance also varies widely in non-diabetic subjects, some of whom are as insulin resistance as diabetic subjects. Therefore, this defect alone cannot account for diabetes.

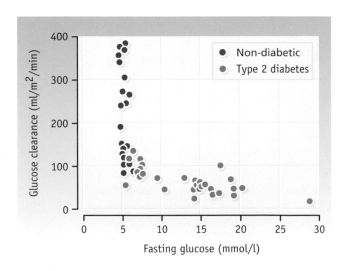

Figure 8.20
The relationship between fasting plasma glucose concentration and glucose metabolic clearance rates (insulin sensitivity) observed during hyperinsulinaemic, glucose-clamp studies in non-diabetic subjects and patients with type 2 diabetes.

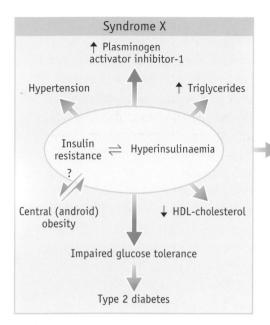

Figure 8.21
The 'insulin resistance syndrome'
('syndrome X').

Insulin resistance is often associated with a clustering of clinical and biochemical features known as metabolic 'syndrome X' or the insulin resistance syndrome. This consists of glucose intolerance, truncal (central) obesity, hypertension, accelerated atherosclerosis, low serum high density lipoprotein (HDL) cholesterol and high triglyceride and very low density lipoprotein (VLDL) concentrations. This lipid abnormality of low serum HDL cholesterol and high triglyceride levels (serum total and LDL cholesterol concentrations are relatively normal) is characteristic of type 2 diabetes and is also known as 'dyslipidaemia'. Other abnormalities associated with syndrome X are increased concentrations of plasminogen activator inhibitor-1 and fibrinogen which promote coagulation.

Recent studies of neuroendocrine peptides and cytokines suggest a role for these in type 2 diabetes, particularly in animals. Leptin is a protein secreted by adipose tissue that inhibits feeding in animals, possibly by inhibiting neuropeptide Y neurones (which stimulate feeding) in the hypothalamus. Leptin defects could therefore give rise to overeating; mutations in the leptin gene are present in the *ob/ob* genetically obese/diabetic mouse, and mutations in the hypothalamic leptin receptor occur in the diabetic, obese and insulin resistant *db/db* mouse and *fa/fa* rat. Adipose tissue also secretes the cytokine, tumour necrosis factor α (TNFα). TNFα causes insulin resistance by inhibiting the tyrosine kinase activity of the insulin receptor and decreasing the expression of the glucose transporter, GLUT-4.

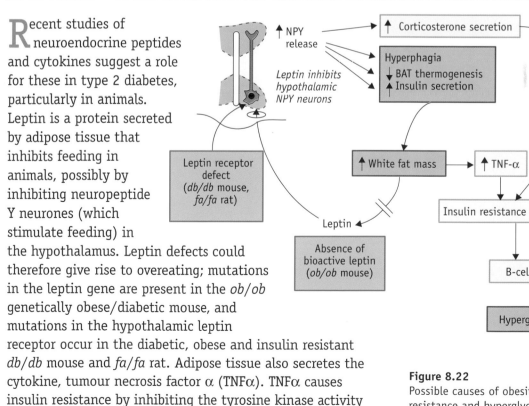

Figure 8.22
Possible causes of obesity, insulin resistance and hyperglycaemia in the *ob/ob*, and *db/db* mouse and *fa/fa* rat.

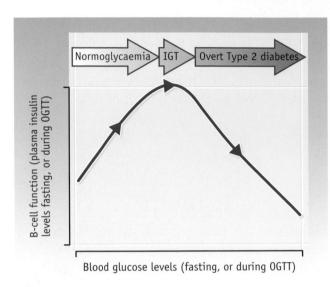

Figure 8.23
The 'Starling curve of the pancreas'.

The relative importance of insulin resistance or B-cell failure in type 2 diabetes and whether one defect appears before the other in the natural history of the disease is uncertain and much disputed. Some studies indicate that insulin resistance appears before impaired insulin secretion. The resultant hyperglycaemia stimulates insulin secretion, leading to hyperinsulinaemia so as to compensate and resist blood glucose increases (IGT phase). Because of B-cell defects, maximal insulin secretory capacity is eventually reached; beyond that point—which corresponds to impaired glucose tolerance (IGT)—insulin secretion declines and overt diabetes results. This bell-shaped curve is known as the 'Starling curve of the pancreas'.

Chapter 9
Other types of diabetes

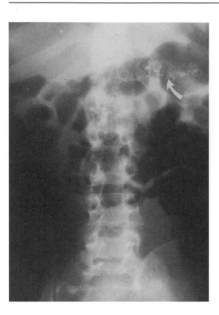

Many pancreatic diseases cause diabetes. Chronic pancreatitis is associated with diabetes, and is mostly due to alcoholism in Western countries. Intraductal protein plugs subsequently calcify, with cyst formation, inflammation and fibrosis. One-third of patients require insulin but ketoacidosis is rare.

Figure 9.1
Plain abdominal radiograph showing pancreatic calcification due to chronic pancreatitis.

Genetic (primary) haemochromatosis is an inborn error of metabolism (autosomal recessive) associated with increased iron absorption and tissue deposition of iron, notably in the liver, islets, skin and pituitary gonadotrophs. The classical clinical triad is skin pigmentation ('bronzed diabetes'), cirrhosis and glucose intolerance, with diabetes (mostly insulin-dependent) in about 25% of the total number of cases. Secondary haemochromatosis can occur in patients requiring frequent transfusions, e.g. for β-thalassaemia.

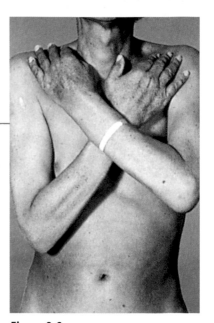

Figure 9.2
Bronzed pigmentation of the skin in a patient with genetic haemochromatosis.

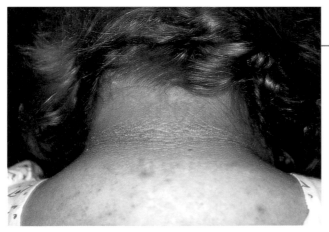

Figure 9.3
Acanthosis nigricans. Nape of the neck of a 26-year-old woman with the type A syndrome.

There are several rare genetic and acquired syndromes of severe insulin resistance. Type A syndrome almost always affects women, in whom there is insulin resistance, manifest by hyperinsulinaemia, hyperandrogenism, and acanthosis nigricans, an area of hyperpigmented skin. Many of these patients have mutations in the insulin receptor.

Leprechaunism is a rare congenital syndrome (growth retardation, dysmorphic facies, lipoatrophy, acanthosis nigricans, insulin resistance) in which there are also mutations in the insulin receptor.

Figure 9.4
Leprechaunism.

In type B syndrome, IgG autoantibodies are directed at the insulin receptor and block and/or mimic insulin action. Most patients are women, often of African descent.

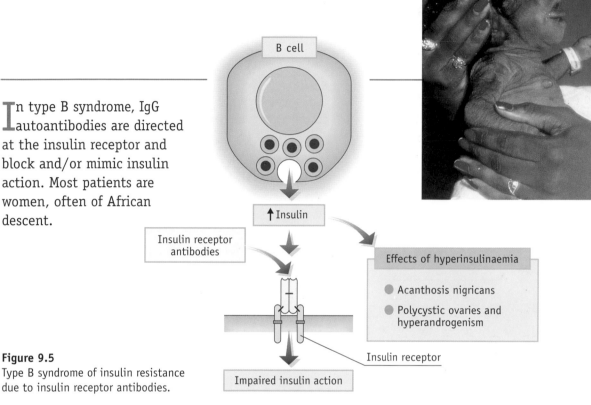

Figure 9.5
Type B syndrome of insulin resistance due to insulin receptor antibodies.

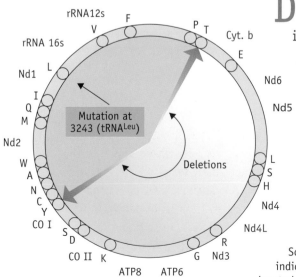

Diabetes or impaired glucose tolerance (IGT) are associated with several syndromes due to mutations in mitochondrial DNA (maternally inherited), the main clinical features of these syndromes are neurological abnormalities. For example, a point mutation in mtDNA encoding the transfer RNA for the amino acid leucine leads to maternally transmitted diabetes with sensorineural deafness, and/or MELAS syndrome (myopathy, encephalopathy, lactic acidosis and stroke-like episodes).

Figure 9.6
Schematic representation of mitochondrial DNA (mtDNA). Circles indicate the 22 tRNA genes. The mutation at the base pair 3243 is located in the gene for tRNA Leu (arrow). Deletions in Pearson's and Kearns–Sayre syndromes may encompass the larger part of the genome.

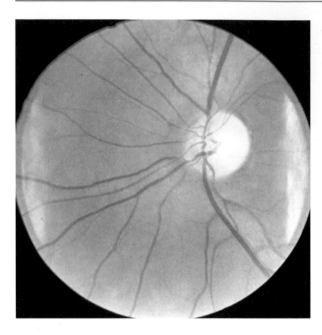

Wolfram syndrome or DIDMOAD is an inherited progressive neurodegenerative disease that comprises diabetes insipidus (DI), insulin-dependent diabetes mellitus (DM), optic atrophy (OA) and sensorineural deafness (D). It has been attributed to a combination of a mtDNA mutation and a defect on chromosome 4.

Figure 9.7
Optic atrophy in a 55-year-old woman with DIDMOAD syndrome.

Insulinopathies are rare genetic conditions, inherited in an autosomal dominant fashion, in which mutations arise in the human insulin gene. The mutations fall into two groups: either leading to insulin with an abnormal structure or a proinsulin intermediate with C peptide still attached. Since the individuals are heterozygous, both normal and abnormal insulin are present in the circulation. Such patients usually display hyperinsulinaemia and varying degrees of glucose intolerance, but a normal response to exogenous insulin.

Name	Amino acid replacement	Designation	Normal codon	Mutant codon	Abnormal secreted product
Insulin Chicago	Phe^{B25} by Leu	Human insulin B25 (Phe→Leu)	TTC	TTG	$[Leu^{B25}]$ insulin*
Insulin Los Angeles	Phe^{B24} by Ser	Human insulin B24 (Phe→Ser)	TTC	TCC	$[Ser^{B24}]$ insulin*
Insulin Wakayama	Val^{A3} by Leu	Human insulin A3 (Val→Leu)	GTG	TTG	$[Leu^{A3}]$ insulin*
Proinsulin Tokyo	Arg^{65} by His	Human proinsulin 65 (Arg→His)	CGC	CAC	des-Arg^{31}, Arg^{32}-$[His^{65}]$ proinsulin†
Proinsulin Boston	Arg^{65} by ?‡	Human proinsulin 65 (Arg→?)‡	?‡	?‡	des-Arg^{31}, Arg^{32}-[Xxx] proinsulin‡

*   Abnormal insulin

†   Abnormal intermediate of proinsulin processing in which the C peptide remains joined to the insulin A chain due to an amino acid replacement at the processing site.

‡   The nature of the secreted product is the same as that for Proinsulin Tokyo, but the amino acid replacement is not yet known.

Figure 9.8
Some known examples of mutant human insulin genes and associated abnormal insulins.

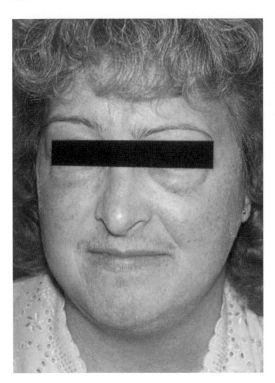

Endocrine conditions associated with diabetes mellitus include Cushing's syndrome, i.e. glucocorticoid excess of any cause. Diabetes, usually non-insulin-dependent, affects about 25% of these patients. Glucocorticoids stimulate hepatic gluconeogenesis and inhibit glucose uptake into peripheral tissues.

Figure 9.9
This 43-year-old woman was referred to the diabetic clinic with glycosuria. Oral glucose tolerance testing revealed IGT. Cushing's syndrome, suggested by her rounded, plethoric face and facial hirsutes and truncal obesity, was diagnosed.

Acromegaly, growth hormone excess due to an anterior pituitary tumour, causes a non-insulin-dependent type of diabetes or IGT, each in about 30% of cases. Growth hormone induces insulin resistance in both liver and peripheral tissue. Glucose intolerance returns to normal with effective lowering of growth hormone levels.

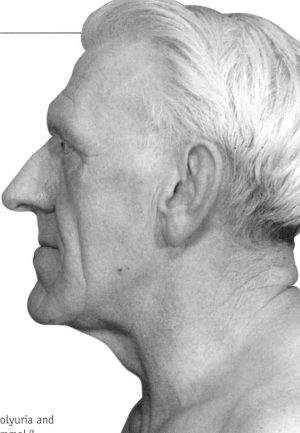

Figure 9.10
Acromegaly and diabetes. This man presented with thirst and polyuria and was found to have a fasting blood glucose concentration of 11 mmol/l.

HANDBOOK OF DIABETES *2ND EDITION*

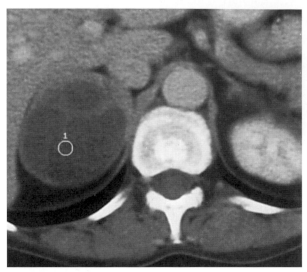

Figure 9.11
Large phaeochromocytoma arising from the right adrenal gland (targeted) in a 49-year-old woman.

Phaeochromocytomas are tumours arising from the chromaffin cells of the sympathetic nervous system, usually in the adrenal medulla. They secrete adrenaline and/or noradrenaline, and sometimes dopamine. Up to 75% of patients have IGT. Catecholamines have several anti-insulin effects, including inhibiting insulin secretion, stimulating glucagon secretion, stimulating liver and muscle glycogenolysis and adipose tissue lipolysis, and causing resistance to insulin-stimulated glucose uptake by a post-receptor mechanism.

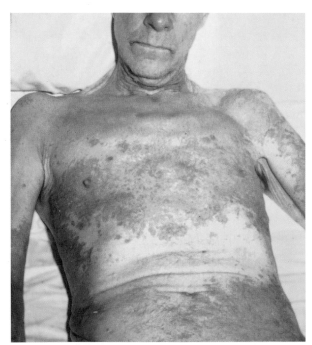

Figure 9.12
Necrolytic migratory erythema characteristic of the glucagonoma syndrome.

Glucagonomas are A-cell tumours of the islets. They are slow growing but usually malignant. The most striking clinical feature is a characteristic rash, termed necrolytic migratory erythema. Diabetes is caused by the gluconeogenesis induced by glucagon.

Chapter 10
Assessing control in diabetes

Diabetic control is the extent to which metabolism in a patient differs from normal. Measurement has traditionally focused on glucose, thus 'strict' or 'good' blood glucose control refers to the maintenance of near-normal blood glucose concentrations throughout the day. However, many blood metabolite levels are abnormal in diabetes, such as ketone bodies, amino acids, lactate, fatty acids and so on. There are many indices of control; common measures are blood and urine glucose concentrations, measures of integrated blood glucose levels such as glycated haemoglobin and urine ketone concentrations.

Index	Main clinical use
Urine glucose	Only crude index of BG, 'last resort' in type 2 diabetes

Blood glucose
  Fasting
  Diurnal/circadian profiles
	
	Correlated with mean daily BG and HbA1 in type 2 diabetes
	Self-monitoring of BG, hospital assessment

Glycated haemoglobin	Glycaemic control (mean) over preceding 1–3 months
Glycated serum protein e.g. 'fructosamine'	Glycaemic control (mean) over preceding 2 weeks
Urine ketones	Insulin deficiency, warning of DKA

Other blood metabolites/hormones
  cholesterol
  triglyceride
	
	Cardiovascular risk factor
	Cardiovascular risk factor

Figure 10.1
Some indices of diabetic control. BG, blood glucose; DKA, diabetic ketoacidosis.

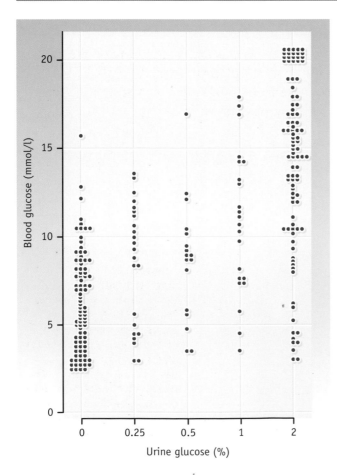

Glycosuria occurs when the blood glucose levels exceed the renal threshold for glucose, 10 mmol/l on average. However, urine glucose testing is an unreliable way of assessing blood glucose control because the renal threshold varies between and within patients, fluid intake affects urine glucose concentrations, and the result does not reflect the blood glucose at the time of testing but over the time that urine accumulated in the bladder. A negative urine test, for example, cannot distinguish between hypoglycaemia, normoglycaemia and moderate hyperglycaemia.

Figure 10.2
Blood glucose concentrations corresponding to various urine glucose tests (0–2%) in diabetic children.

Urine glucose testing remains a reasonable option in stable type 2 diabetic patients and in those unable or unwilling to perform blood glucose tests, but should be supplemented by regular blood tests.

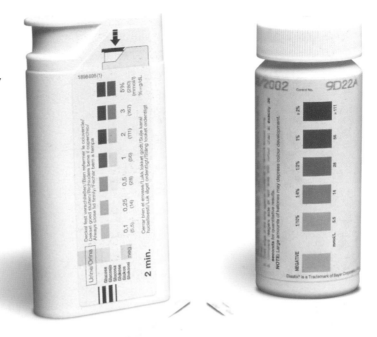

Figure 10.3
Urine testing strips.

Blood glucose levels fluctuate widely in type 1 diabetic subjects and are fairly unpredictable. Thus, single blood glucose measurements give little or no information about overall control. In type 2 diabetes, blood glucose levels are more stable from day to day, and a single blood glucose sample (particularly when fasting) gives a reasonable estimate of control.

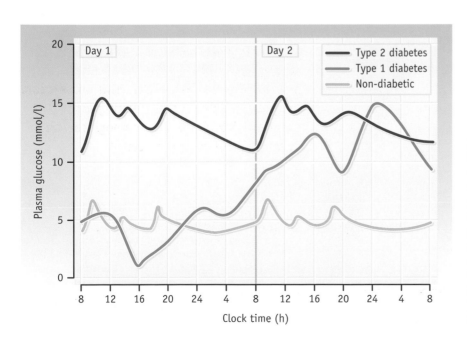

Figure 10.4
Schematic representation of variations in plasma glucose concentrations over 2 days in a non-diabetic person, a type 1 diabetic patient (wide swings in glucose levels with little day-to-day consistency) and type 2 diabetes patient (similar profile to non-diabetic subject but at a higher level and with greater postprandial peaks; fairly consistent from day to day).

HANDBOOK OF DIABETES *2ND EDITION*

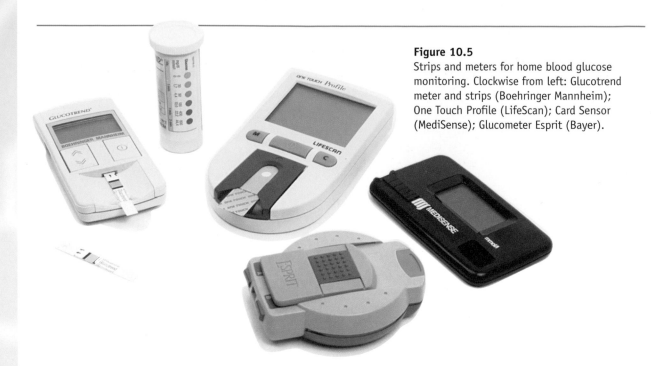

Figure 10.5
Strips and meters for home blood glucose monitoring. Clockwise from left: Glucotrend meter and strips (Boehringer Mannheim); One Touch Profile (LifeScan); Card Sensor (MediSense); Glucometer Esprit (Bayer).

The best assessment of glucose control is provided by timed measurements of blood glucose concentration throughout the day. Self-monitoring of capillary blood glucose by patients at home using glucose-oxidase-impregnated reagent strips is now an integral part of intensified insulin treatment. Strips usually contain glucose oxidase and peroxidase and a chromagen that changes colour in proportion to the glucose concentration. The colour can be assessed in comparison with a chart or measured in a reflectance meter. Newer, electrochemically-based strips generate a current rather than a colour change. Meters are particularly useful for patients with colour vision defects due to retinopathy or other causes.

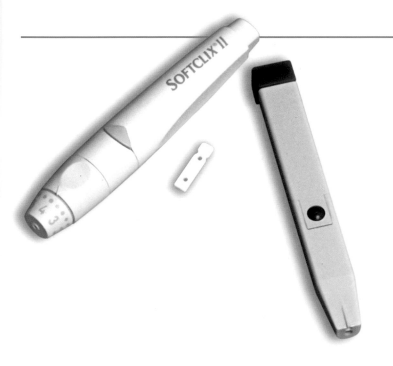

Several devices containing a spring-loaded lancet are available for obtaining a blood sample. The fingers are the usual site of sampling.

Figure 10.6
Devices for automatic finger-pricking. Left, the Softclix II (Boehringer Mannheim); right, the Penlet II (LifeScan). These are spring-loaded devices in which the lancet is released at the press of a button.

Target blood glucose levels	
Before meals	4–7 mmol/l
90–120 min after meals	4–10 mmol/l
Before bedtime snack	7–10 mmol/l
At 0300 h	3.5–7 mmol/l
If blood glucose is usually too high:	
Before breakfast	Increase evening delayed-action insulin
Before lunch	Increase morning short-acting insulin
Before evening meal	Increase morning delayed-action insulin *or* prelunch short-acting insulin
Before bedtime	Increase evening short-acting insulin
If blood glucose is usually too low:	
Before breakfast	Reduce evening delayed-action insulin
Before lunch	Reduce morning short-acting insulin *or* increase mid-morning snack
Before evening meal	Reduce morning delayed-action insulin *or* lunchtime short-acting insulin *or* increase mid-afternoon snack
Before bed	Reduce pre-evening meal short-acting insulin

Figure 10.7

Algorithm for adjusting insulin dosage according to blood glucose results.

Based on the self-monitored blood glucose values, the insulin dose and food intake of a patient can be adjusted to optimise control. Algorithms, or rules, can be helpful in suggesting insulin dose changes in response to high or low blood glucose levels at particular times of the day.

Glycated haemoglobin (GHb) (also known as glycosylated haemoglobin or glycohaemoglobin) is a measure of the integrated blood glucose control over the preceding 2–3 months, but with extra weighting for the one month before blood sampling. The major component is HbA_{1c} which is formed by the slow, non-enzymatic attachment of glucose to the N-terminal β-chain of haemoglobin, followed by a rearrangement to form a stable ketoamine derivative of haemoglobin.

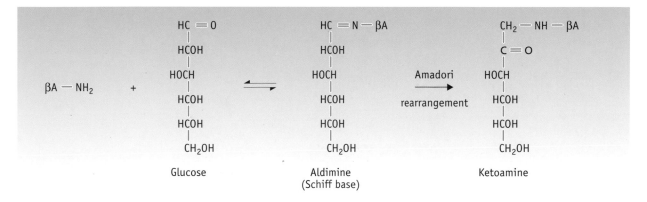

Figure 10.8

The mechanism of glycated haemoglobin (HbA_{1c}) formation. Glucose forms a Schiff base linkage to the N-terminal valine of the β-chain of haemoglobin, which rearranges to the stable ketoamine product.

HANDBOOK OF DIABETES *2ND EDITION*

GHb can be measured by several methods in the laboratory, including gel electrophoresis, high-performance liquid chromatography and affinity chromatography. An immunoassay-based bench-top analyser (DCA 2000, Bayer Diagnostics) is available for GHb assay in the diabetes clinic, doctor's office and similar settings. The reference range for HbA_{1c} in non-diabetic subjects is about 4–6%, but normal ranges are not interchangeable between laboratories because of assay variations and the difficulty of standardisation.

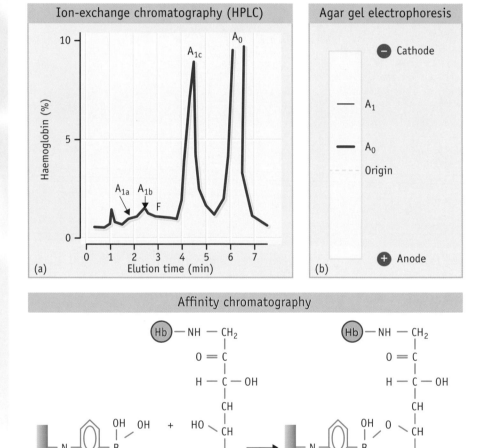

Figure 10.9
Three commonly used methods for glycated haemoglobin analysis. (a) Ion-exchange chromatography, (b) agar gel electrophoresis and (c) affinity chromatography.

HANDBOOK OF DIABETES *2ND EDITION*

Serum 'fructosamine' is a measure of glycated serum proteins, mostly albumin, and is an index of control over the previous 2–3 weeks, the lifetime of albumin. Colorimetric assays for fructosamine are based on glycated protein acting as a reducing agent in alkaline solution. The methods are suitable for automated analysers. The reference range for non-diabetic subjects is about 205–285 µmol/l. The test is an alternative to GHb, and generally correlates well with GHb, but is perhaps especially useful for assessing changes in control over short periods, such as in pregnancy. At present, GHb is the more commonly used index of long-term glycaemic control.

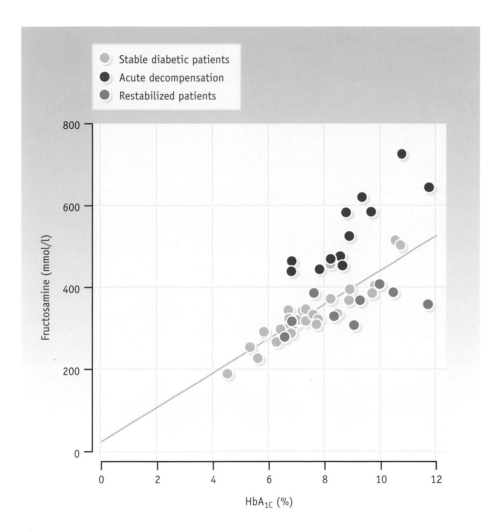

Figure 10.10
Correlation of serum fructosamine and HbA$_{1c}$ in diabetic patients. The correlation is best in stable diabetic patients and worst in those whose control has changed markedly in recent weeks.

Raised urinary ketones reflect severe insulin deficiency, and either indicate or warn against impending ketoacidosis. Ketone tests are based on nitroprusside and mainly detect acetoacetate and acetone rather than 3-hydroxybutyrate, which is quantitatively the most important ketone body. Blood 3-hydroxybutyrate levels are not routinely measured, but reagent strips for this ketone body are now becoming available.

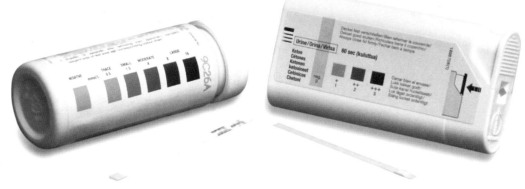

Figure 10.11
Urine ketone strips.

Chapter 11
Management of
type 1 diabetes

Optimised or intensive insulin treatment

- Physiological insulin regimen
- Assessment of control
- Dosage adjustment
- Diet and exercise
- Diabetes education

Figure 11.1
Optimised or intensive insulin treatment.

Modern 'optimised' treatment of type 1 diabetic patients involves much more than insulin injections. Management encompasses a package of measures which includes 'physiological' insulin injection regimens, assessment of control (usually by home blood glucose monitoring and hospital tests of control), insulin dosage adjustments, a healthy diet and adequate exercise, and diabetes education.

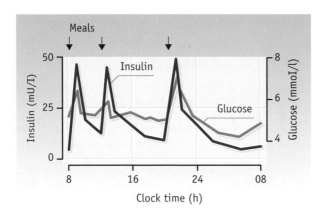

Figure 11.2
24-hour profiles of blood insulin and glucose concentrations in non-diabetic subjects.

The philosophy of insulin replacement is to mimic with injections the insulin secretion pattern in the non-diabetic person, so-called physiological insulin delivery. Here, insulin is secreted at two rates: a slow basal secretion throughout the 24 hours, which gives rise to low blood insulin levels between meals and during the night, and an augmented rate at mealtimes. The basal insulin concentration is sufficient to suppress liver glucose output and the bolus, postprandial concentration stimulates glucose uptake into the periphery.

Insulin injection regimens therefore use short-acting (unmodified) insulin to simulate normal mealtime insulin levels, and delayed-action insulin to provide a background concentration of insulin. This is sometimes called the 'basal-bolus' strategy.

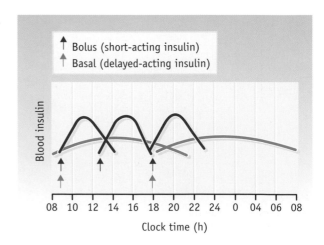

Figure 11.3
'Basal-bolus' insulin regimen.

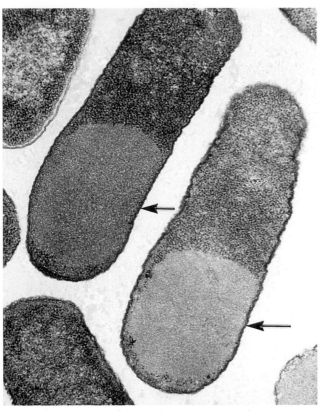

Figure 11.4
Transmission electron micrograph of *Escherichia coli* cells showing expressed chimeric promoter–insulin (arrows).

Until the 1980s, insulin was extracted and purified from the pancreas of cows and pigs. Animal insulins are still in use, but are being superseded by human-sequence insulin. In many European countries, and in North America, human insulin is now the main species of insulin in routine clinical use. It is usually manufactured by recombinant DNA technology, i.e. by insertion of synthesised genes for the insulin A-chain and B-chain, or a proinsulin-like precursor gene, into *Escherichia coli* bacteria or yeast cells. Fermentation results in large amounts of protein which can be converted to insulin and purified.

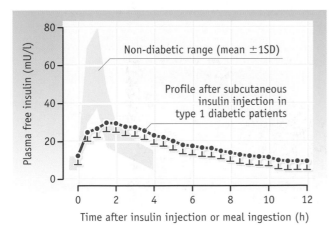

Figure 11.5
Plasma insulin concentration in response to a mixed meal in non-diabetic subjects (shaded area) and in type 1 diabetic patients after subcutaneous injection of insulin.

Short-acting insulin, also known as regular or soluble insulin, consists of unmodified insulin in solution at neutral pH. The duration of peak action is about 1–3 hours, so it is normally injected subcutaneously about 30 minutes before a main meal, when the peak of blood insulin corresponds to the blood glucose rise after the meal.

HANDBOOK OF DIABETES *2ND EDITION*

Intermediate-acting or delayed-action insulins are of two main types. Isophane is an insoluble suspension of insulin made by combining insulin with the highly basic protein, protamine, with zinc ions at neutral pH. It is also called NPH (neutral protamine Hagedorn, after the Hagedorn laboratories in Copenhagen where it was developed in the 1940s). Lente insulins are insoluble insulins made by adding excess zinc ions to insulin. Both isophane and lente have a duration of about 8–12 hours after subcutaneous injection. A variation of lente called ultralente with larger, more insoluble crystals has a duration of more than 24 hours when made from beef insulin, but its human formulation is similar in duration to isophane and lente insulins. Long-acting insulins which are soluble in the vial but precipitate subcutaneously on injection are being manufactured by protein engineering techniques, for example insulin glargine (HOE 901, Aventis), which is expected to be marketed in the year 2000.

Insulin class	Time of action (h)			Species or origin
	Onset	Peak	Duration	
Short-acting insulins				
Monomeric	<0.5	0.5–2.5	3.0–4.5	Synthetic
Short-acting (soluble, regular)	0.2–0.5	1.0–3.0	4.0–8.0	Human, porcine, bovine
Intermediate-acting (delayed-action) insulins				
Isophane (NPH)	1.0–2.0	4.0–6.0	8.0–12.0	Human, porcine, bovine
Lente	1.0–2.0	4.0–8.0	8.0–14	Human, porcine, bovine
	1.0–3.0	5.0–10	10–24	Porcine, bovine
Long-acting insulins				
Ultralente	2.0–3.0	4.0–8.0	8.0–14	Human
	2.0–4.0	6.0–12	12–28	Bovine
Insulin glargine (* = plateau)	3.0–5.0	6.0–24*	~ 24	Synthetic

Figure 11.6
Duration of action of insulins.

Pharmacokinetic studies in normal subjects and type 1 diabetic patients have shown that insulin glargine activity is essentially peakless, and 50% lower and of two-fold longer duration than human isophane insulin. A recent 28-week randomised trial in type 1 diabetic subjects treated with short-acting insulin plus bedtime glargine or short-acting insulin plus once or twice daily NPH resulted in a fasting plasma glucose level about 1.3 mmol/l lower and a more than 50% reduction in the frequency of hypoglycaemia (< 2.0 mmol/l) on the glargine regimen. Similar results with type 2 diabetic subjects suggest that this new insulin may benefit patients with both type 1 and 2 diabetes.

A variety of pre-mixed or 'biphasic' insulins are also available, where set ratios of short-acting and NPH insulin have been mixed by the manufacturer. A 30% short-acting/70% NPH mixture is the most common formulation.

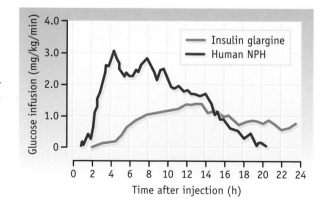

Figure 11.7
Median glucose infusion rate in euglycaemic clamp (a measure of hypoglycaemic activity) in normal subjects after s.c. injection of insulin glargine or human NPH.

'Monomeric' insulin analogues have been introduced in recent years in order to speed the absorption of subcutaneously-injected insulin. At pharmacological concentration, insulin is self-associated as a hexamer (a group of six molecules), which is too large to be absorbed into the circulation when injected into the subcutaneous tissue. Absorption is slow because of the time needed for diffusion and dilution to occur, which causes dissociation into dimers and monomers that are small enough to be absorbed.

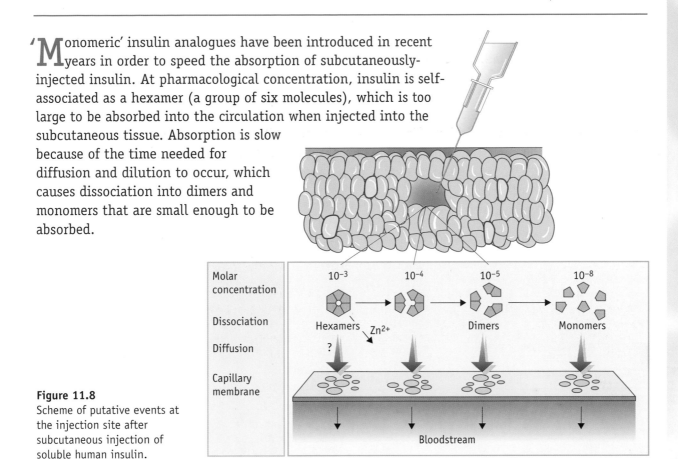

Figure 11.8
Scheme of putative events at the injection site after subcutaneous injection of soluble human insulin.

Using genetic and protein engineering techniques, changes are made in the amino acid sequence of insulin that reduce the tendency to self-associate, e.g. by charge repulsion. The first monomeric insulin to be introduced was lispro insulin (Humalog, Eli Lilly) where the B28 lysine and B29 proline residues of native insulin are reversed (B28 Lys, B29 Pro insulin). Aspart insulin (Novo Nordisk) is another monomeric insulin currently undergoing trial.

Strategy	Example
Charge repulsion	B9 Asp (Ser), B12 Glu (Val), B28 Asp (Pro)
Steric hindrance	B12 Ile (Val)
Hydrophilic into hydrophobic interfaces	B16 Glu (Tyr), B17, Gln (Leu)
Removal of cation metal-binding sites	B10 Asp (His), B10 Thr (His)
Mimicking IGF-1 structure	B28 Lys (Pro), B29 Pro (Lys)

Figure 11.9
Strategies for the manufacture of insulin analogues that have reduced self-association and therefore faster absorption.

HANDBOOK OF DIABETES *2ND EDITION*

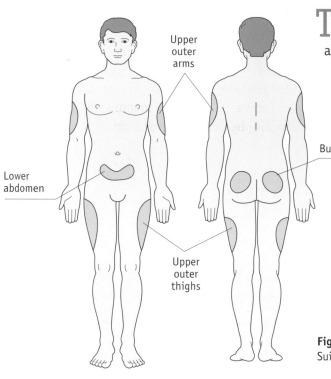

The recommended sites for insulin injection are the subcutaneous tissue of the lower abdomen, upper outer thighs, upper outer arms and the buttocks. Disposable plastic syringes with a fine needle can be re-used for several injections, until the needle becomes blunt.

Upper outer arms

Buttocks

Lower abdomen

Upper outer thighs

Figure 11.10
Suitable sites for subcutaneous insulin injection.

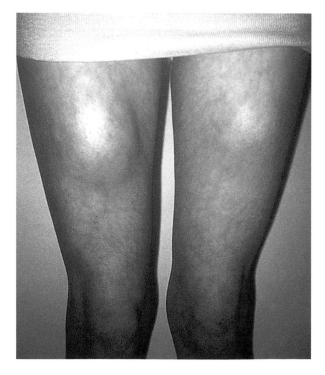

The rate of insulin absorption varies at different sites—fastest in the abdomen and slowest in the thigh and buttocks. Injection into the same subcutaneous site in the long term may give rise to an accumulation of fat, lipohypertrophy, which is due to the local trophic action of insulin. The site of insulin injection therefore ideally should be rotated within a given anatomical area to prevent lipohypertrophy—which can be unsightly and also increases the variability of absorption.

Figure 11.11
Lipohypertrophy.

HANDBOOK OF DIABETES *2ND EDITION*

A nother local reaction to insulin injection is lipoatrophy. This unsightly hollowing of the subcutaneous fat is thought to be due to local deposition of insulin-IgG immune complexes. With modern, highly purified insulins which do not induce a significant immune response, lipoatrophy is hardly ever seen.

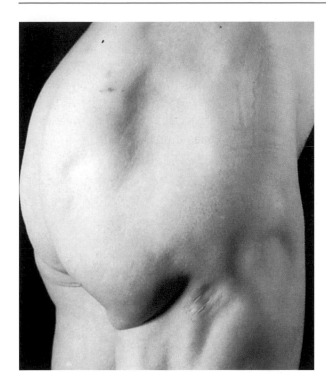

Figure 11.12
Extensive areas of lipoatrophy in a 39-year-old woman treated for over 20 years with various 'impure' insulin preparations.

I nsulin 'pens' have become a popular option for injection therapy in recent years. The insulin is contained in a reservoir in the pen-shaped barrel which also incorporates a fine needle. The required dosage is achieved by a series of presses on a plunger, before inserting the needle or dialled up. The many advantages of insulin pens include convenience and ease of injection, less painful injection (because the needle remains sharp for longer, as it is not reinserted through the rubber diaphragm of an insulin vial), and good patient acceptance, thereby encouraging multiple injection regimens.

Figure 11.13
Insulin injection 'pens'.
From left to right: the OptiPen Pro 1
(Aventis Pharma); the Autopen (Owen Mumford);
the B-D Pen (Becton Dickinson); two examples
of the NovoPen 3 (Novo Nordisk); the HumaPen (Eli Lilly).

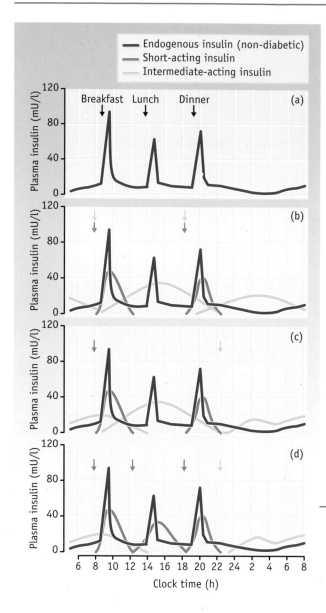

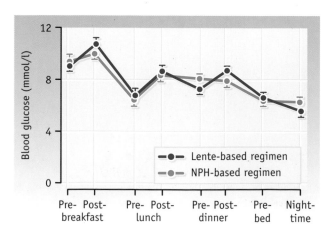

A popular insulin regimen for type 1 diabetic patients involves twice daily injections of short- and intermediate-acting insulin given before breakfast and the evening meal. However, the action of intermediate-acting insulin tends to wane after about 0300 hours when it is injected at about 1800 hours, resulting in high pre-breakfast blood glucose levels. Delaying the evening injection of isophane or lente insulin until bedtime improves fasting blood glucose concentrations.

Figure 11.14
Schematic plasma insulin profiles from various insulin treatment regimens using short- and intermediate-acting (isophane and lente) insulins, compared with: (a) the plasma insulin profile from a non-diabetic subject eating three meals a day; (b) twice-daily mixed injections; (c) the effect of moving the evening intermediate-acting insulin to bedtime; and (d) a basal bolus regimen of short-acting insulin before each mean meal and intermediate-acting insulin at bedtime.

In theory, it is not advisable to mix short-acting and lente insulin in the same syringe because some of the excess zinc ions in lente complexes with unmodified insulin, converting it to more lente. This does not occur with isophane. However, in clinical practice the glycaemic control achieved by isophane and lente-based regimens is almost identical, even when no particular precautions are taken over mixing them with short-acting insulin.

Figure 11.15
The glycaemic equivalence of regimens based on isophane or lente insulins. Mean ± SEM blood glucose values from samples collected by patients at home on filter paper and later analysed in a laboratory.

Experience with insulin lispro is just beginning. Because of the rapid absorption, lispro can be injected immediately before a meal and postprandial glucose levels are significantly reduced compared to regular, short-acting insulin. Because lispro insulin runs out more quickly than does regular short-acting insulin, blood glucose levels before the next meal may be a little higher. Insulin aspart (Novo Nordisk) is another monomeric insulin which is absorbed very rapidly from the site of subcutaneous injection and therefore designed for administration at mealtimes. Clinical trials indicate that there is effective improvement in postprandial glycaemic control with aspart, though night-time blood glucose levels can be higher than with human short-acting insulin. Optimisation of control using these new very short-acting insulin analogues is therefore likely also to require compensatory adjustments of the dosage and timing of basal insulin components such as isophane.

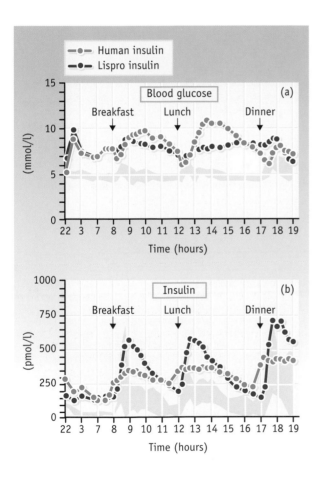

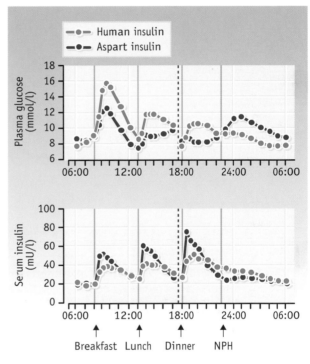

Figure 11.16
Mean ± SD blood glucose and insulin concentrations in 12 subjects with type 1 diabetes treated by human insulin or lispro. NPH was given at bedtime. (Shaded area: non-diabetic responses.)

Figure 11.17
Serum insulin and plasma glucose profile in type 1 diabetic patients treated by insulin aspart or unmodified human insulin.

Alternative insulin delivery systems

Insulin infusion systems can be either 'open-loop', in which basal and prandial insulin infusion rates are preselected by the doctor or patient; or 'closed loop' (the so-called 'artificial endocrine pancreas'), where there is frequent or continuous blood or tissue glucose sensing with computer-regulated feedback control of the insulin delivery, so as to maintain normoglycaemia.

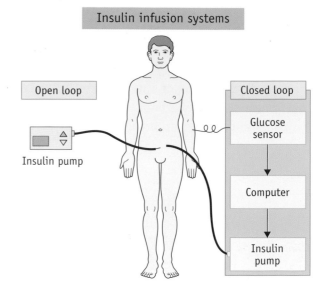

Figure 11.18
Open- and closed-loop insulin delivery systems.

Continuous subcutaneous insulin infusion (CSII) is an open-loop insulin delivery system where a rate-adjustable portable pump is used to infuse insulin into the subcutaneous tissue. Basal insulin delivery with CSII is about 1 U/h in most adults and, unlike delayed-action insulin injections, is constant. Because of this and the preprandial boosts before each main meal, CSII more closely simulates non-diabetic insulin secretory patterns than does conventional injection therapy.

Figure 11.19
Two insulin infusion pumps designed for CSII. (a) Disetronic H-Tron V100 (Disetronic Medical Systems, Burgdorf, Switzerland). (b) MiniMed 506 (MiniMed Technologies, Sylmar, CA, USA).

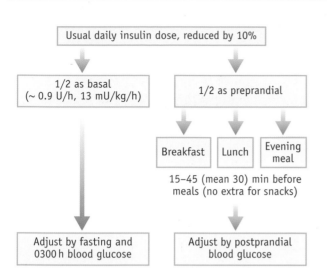

HANDBOOK OF DIABETES *2ND EDITION*

A typical initial strategy for CSII is to administer about half the daily insulin as the basal rate and to divide the remaining half amongst the three main meals. When starting patients on CSII, it is also necessary to provide comprehensive education about pump therapy, blood glucose self-monitoring, dosage adjustments, and corrective action in case of hypoglycaemia, hyperglycaemia or intercurrent illness.

Figure 11.20
An infusion strategy for starting patients on CSII.

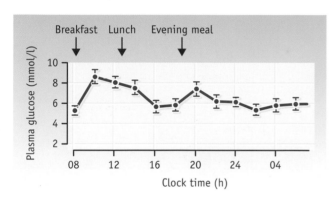

Figure 11.21
Plasma glucose concentrations throughout the day (mean ± SEM) in 30 subjects with type 1 diabetes treated by CSII.

Excellent glycaemic control can be obtained with CSII in most patients, which can be maintained for years, if desired. Short-acting insulin (Velosulin, Humulin S/R, Actrapid) has traditionally been used in the pump reservoir, but first trials with the recently introduced monomeric insulin analogue, lispro (Humalog) indicate that HbA$_{1c}$ is lower using this insulin for CSII and that variability of control may be improved.

- When optimized conventional insulin injection treatment has failed (e.g. in some hypoglycaemia-prone diabetic subjects)
- When the centre has special expertise and experience of CSII
- When the patient prefers CSII (e.g. dislikes multiple injections)
- When the patient has an erratic lifestyle (more flexibility to omit or delay mealtimes)
- Recurrent hypoglycaemia and/or hypoglycaemia unawareness
- Pregnancy or other indication for strict control
- A marked dawn phenomenon (pre-breakfast blood glucose rise)

Figure 11.22
When to consider CSII.

CSII is an alternative form of intensified insulin treatment, but it requires special expertise and facilities. Centres undertaking CSII must provide supervision by experienced staff and, preferably, a 24-hour telephone service for advice about management problems. At the moment, it is used in only selected patients.

Totally implanted insulin pumps are still at an experimental stage and are not used for routine treatment of diabetes. Pumps are generally implanted into a pocket in the subcutaneous tissue of the abdomen with a delivery cannula in the peritoneal cavity. Dosage adjustments can be made with an external electronic communicator. Blood glucose control is very good with implanted pumps, with fewer hypoglycaemic episodes and smaller oscillations than with injection therapy.

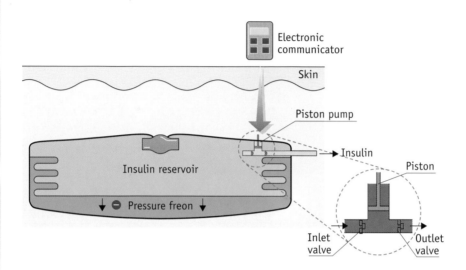

Figure 11.23
Diagrammatic representation of the main features of a programmable implantable medication system. The Freon pressure is less than atmospheric, so that the reservoir is filled without exerting pressure, and any leak would result in drawing of tissue fluid back into the catheter rather than uncontrolled release of insulin into the body. The pump, controlled by an external communicator, is a positive displacement piston design.

HANDBOOK OF DIABETES *2ND EDITION*

Chapter 12
Management of type 2 diabetes

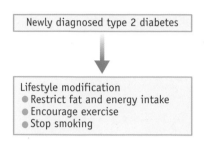

The starting point and mainstay of treatment for type 2 diabetes are diet and other modifications of lifestyle, such as increasing exercise and stopping smoking. Diet is important to reduce weight (up to 80% of type 2 diabetic patients are obese), to lower blood glucose concentrations and increase insulin sensitivity, and to reduce cardiovascular risk factors such as abnormal lipid profiles and hypertension.

Figure 12.1
Management of type 2 diabetes: the initial measures.

The dietary recommendations are essentially the same for type 1 and type 2 diabetes and indeed follow a healthy eating pattern suitable for the entire population. The emphasis should be on a low fat and high carbohydrate intake rather than the avoidance of sugar. Saturated fats should be restricted and monounsaturated fats such as olive oil should be encouraged. Complex high-fibre carbohydrates should be increased in the diet, particularly foods containing soluble fibre such as leaf vegetables, fruits, cereals, roots and pulses. Bread, pasta or potato should be the main part of meals.

Contributions to total energy intake

- Carbohydrate (> 55%)
- Fat (< 30%)
- Protein (10–15%)

- Encourage complex high-fibre carbohydrates
- Limit sucrose (< 25 g/day added; < 50 g/day total)

- Saturated fats < 10% of total energy intake
- Encourage MUFA (olive oil, rapeseed oil)
- Cholesterol < 250 mg/ day (less if dyslipidaemia)

Other recommendations

- Limit salt intake (< 6 g/day; less if hypertension)
- Limit alcohol intake: men < 21 U/week, women < 12 U/week (less if hypertension or dyslipidaemia)
- Avoid 'diabetic' foods

Figure 12.2
Dietary recommendations for patients with type 1 and type 2 diabetes. MUFA, monosaturated fatty acids.

It is normally best to give patients simple dietary guidelines in the form of recommended foods, which are better understood than fat, carbohydrate and protein measures. 'Diabetic' foods containing sorbitol or fructose as a sweetener are not recommended. Sucrose need not be banned from the diabetic diet, and a moderate amount for sweetening is acceptable.

Figure 12.3
Practical food recommendations for patients with type 2 diabetes.

- Quench thirst with water or other sugar-free drinks
- Eat regular meals, avoiding fried and very sugary foods
- Eat plenty of vegetables
- Have cereals, bread, pasta, potato, rice or chapattis as the main part of each meal
- Eat meat, eggs, cheese as a small part of each meal
- Encourage fruit and vegetables, including pulses
- Eat double helpings of vegetables as a part of *every* meal with main meals (The WHO recommendation is 400 g/day, equivalent to 5 × 80 g portions)
- Bread, cereals, pasta or potatoes should form the largest part of each meal or snack
- Meat, cheese, eggs or fish should form only a small part of main meals (e.g. one-quarter of the area of the plate)
- Fish and pulses (e.g. beans) are good alternatives
- For snacks between meals, avoid convenience foods such as biscuits, cake or confectionery (which are high in saturated and *trans*-fatty acids, glucose and salt)
- Use fats and oils that are low in saturated and *trans*-fatty acids (e.g. olive oil) or reduced-fat dairy products
- Avoid spreads on bread
- Drink water, tea, coffee, milk and low-calorie beverages and avoid sugary drinks and alcohol, especially between meals

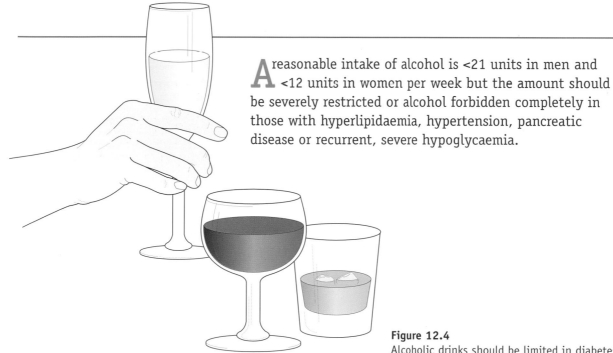

A reasonable intake of alcohol is <21 units in men and <12 units in women per week but the amount should be severely restricted or alcohol forbidden completely in those with hyperlipidaemia, hypertension, pancreatic disease or recurrent, severe hypoglycaemia.

Figure 12.4
Alcoholic drinks should be limited in diabetes.

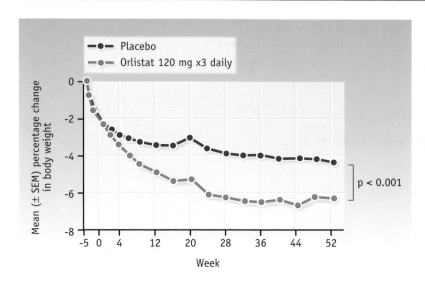

There are few effective, safe and ethically acceptable anti-obesity drugs at present. Orlistat (Xenical®, tetrahydrolipstatin). It acts locally in the gastrointestinal tract where it blocks enzymatic digestion of triglyceride by inhibiting pancreatic lipase), and thus prevents absorption of up to 30% of ingested fat. Sibutramine is a monoamine (serotonin and noradrenaline) reuptake inhibitor which has a central effect and may also be a useful tool in obesity management.

Figure 12.5
Effect of Orlistat in type 2 diabetic patients.

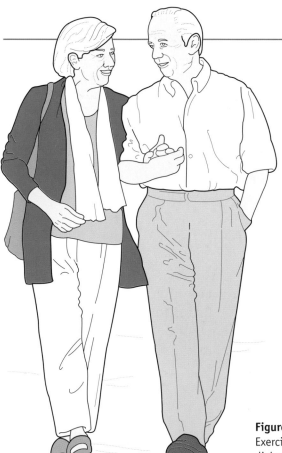

Exercise should be tailored for the individual patient but simple advice might include moderate exercise as part of the daily schedule e.g. walking for 30–60 minutes per day (preferably an extra 30–60 minutes), and using stairs rather than lifts. Exercise does not usually cause hypoglycaemia in type 2 diabetic patients (in contrast to type 1 patients), and therefore extra carbohydrate is generally unnecessary.

Figure 12.6
Exercise is an important part of the management of type 2 diabetic patients.

HANDBOOK OF DIABETES 2ND EDITION

Diet and exercise are sufficient to achieve adequate glycaemic control in only about 10–20% of type 2 diabetic subjects, otherwise an oral hypoglycaemic agent is generally introduced. The long established, first-line drugs are sulphonylureas, which stimulate insulin secretion, and the biguanide, metformin, which increases insulin action and inhibits liver gluconeogenesis. Sulphonylureas are often used in non-obese patients where the main defect is thought to be impaired insulin secretion, while metformin is useful for obese patients who have marked insulin resistance. Another reason for using metformin in obese subjects is that it may also decrease appetite and encourage weight loss.

Agent	Examples
Sulphonylureas	Acetohexamide*, chlorpropamide*, glibenclamide, gliclazide, glipizide, gliquidone, tolazamide, tolbutamide*, glimepiride
Non-sulphonylurea secretagogues	Repaglinide
Biguanides	Metformin
Alpha-glucoside inhibitors	Acarbose
Thiazolidinediones	Troglitazone, rosiglitazone, pioglitazone
Insulin	Premixed insulin: short-acting/isophane
Combination therapy	Insulin + sulphonylurea; insulin + metformin

* First-generation sulphonylureas.
Glibenclamide is known in the USA as glyburide.

Figure 12.7
Current drug therapies for type 2 diabetes.

Metformin in type 2 diabetes
• Suitable for obese, insulin-resistant subjects
• Encourages weight loss
• Gastrointestinal side effects in some
• Lactic acidosis a rare complication

Figure 12.8
Metformin in type 2 diabetes.

The main side-effects of metformin are nausea and diarrhoea, which occur in about 25% of cases and are minimised by taking the drug with meals and at a low starting dose. Lactic acidosis is a rare but potentially fatal complication of metformin use, and the drug should not be given to patients with renal, hepatic, cardiac or respiratory failure.

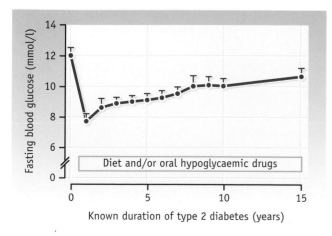

Figure 12.9
Gradually worsening glycaemic control in type 2 diabetic subjects.

Oral agents may fail to control blood glucose levels after a period of apparent success ('secondary failure') because of poor compliance or worsening B-cell function and/or insulin resistance. In these cases, combination therapy of metformin plus a sulphonylurea or addition of an α-glucosidase inhibitor is usually tried. Most patients ultimately require insulin.

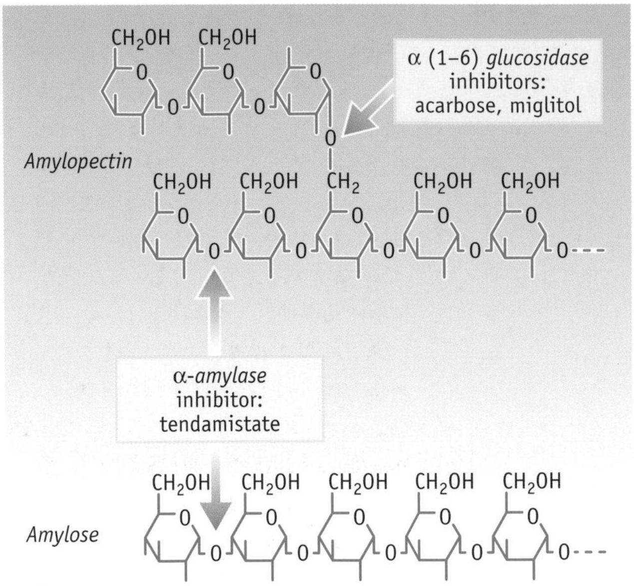

Alpha-glucosidase inhibitors such as acarbose delay carbohydrate absorption by inhibiting disaccharidase enzymes in the gut, responsible for carbohydrate digestion. The drug preferentially lowers postprandial glucose levels. The side-effects are flatulence, abdominal bloating and diarrhoea.

Figure 12.10
Hydrolysis of starch, showing site of side-chain cleavage (α (1–6) glucosidase) that is inhibited by acarbose and miglitol.

Newer oral agents include glimepiride which is a once-daily sulphonylurea which also has an 'extrapancreatic', insulin-sparing action. It has a low risk of hypoglycaemia, perhaps because of its rapid on-off binding to the B-cell. In some countries, extended release preparations of sulphonylureas are available, for example glipizide GITS (Gastrointestinal Therapeutic System). Repaglinide is a fast-acting, short-duration non-sulphonylurea insulin secretagogue, used as a 'prandial glucose regulator'; i.e. it is designed to minimise mealtime blood glucose peaks (see Epidemiology and aetiology of type 2 diabetes, p. 47). Other non-sulphonylurea prandial glucose regulators which are undergoing clinical trial include nateglinide, which is structurally dissimilar to repaglinide.

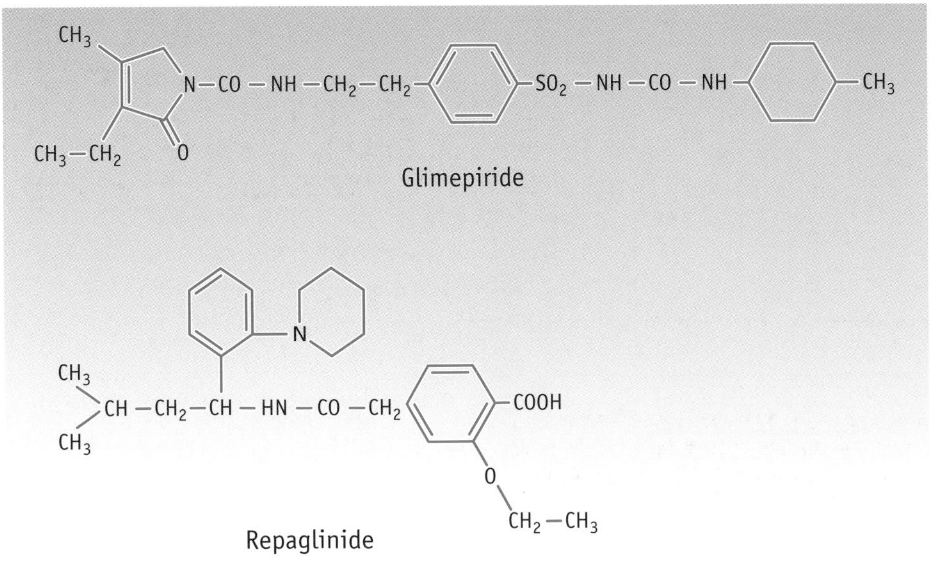

Figure 12.11
Newer oral hypoglycaemic agents.

The crucial importance of insulin resistance in the pathophysiology of type 2 diabetes has led to the recent development of novel agents which potentiate insulin action. Thiazolidinediones bind to the peroxisome proliferator-activated receptor-γ (PPAR-γ), a nuclear receptor involved in the regulation of key genes in adipose tissue and muscle. The first to be introduced into clinical practice was troglitazone in 1997. Troglitazone has been associated with severe hepatic damage in a few cases, and, at the time of writing, it has been withdrawn from clinical use in the UK, but remains available in the USA. Frequent liver function tests are currently recommended (monthly serum alanine aminotransferase levels for the first 8 months of treatment and at regular intervals thereafter). Other thiazolidinediones include rosiglitazone and pioglitazone. Rosiglitazone is the most potent of the thiazolidinediones. In clinical trials to date, no hepatotoxicity has been observed with this agent. In common with other 'glitazones', rosiglitazone improves blood glucose control and reduces hyperinsulinaemia by reducing insulin resistance in type 2 diabetes. Serum triglyceride and free fatty acid concentrations are also reduced by thiazolidinediones treatment.

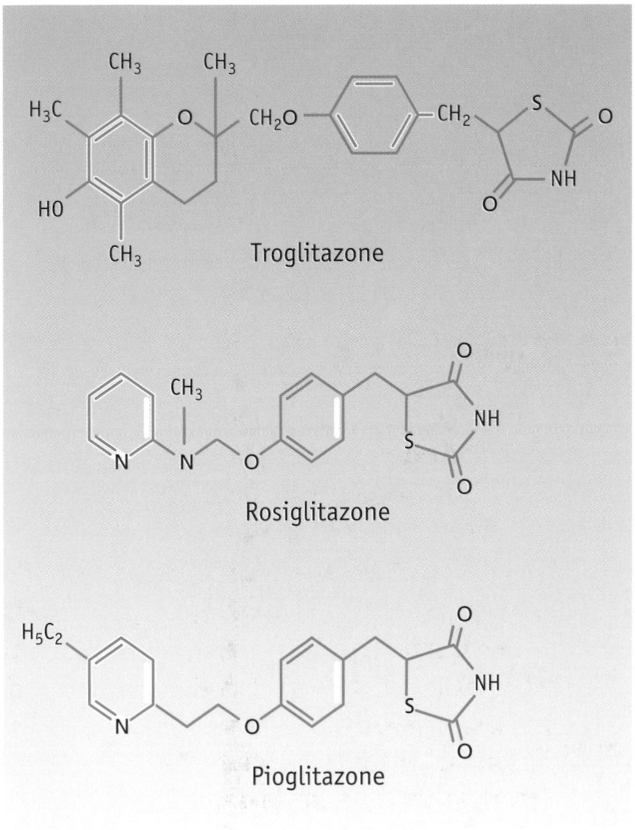

Figure 12.12
Chemical structures of some thiazolidinediones.

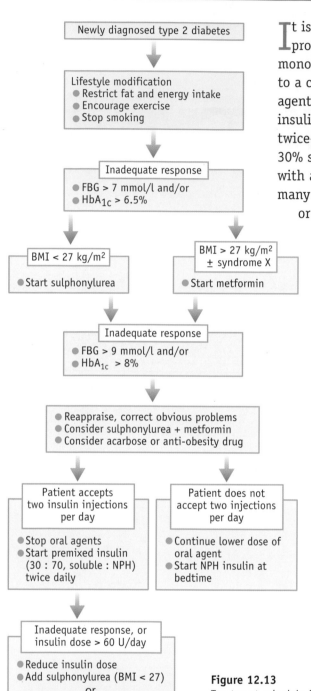

It is common for many type 2 diabetic patients to progress from treatment by diet alone to monotherapy with an oral hypoglycaemic agent, then to a combination of two, and sometimes three, oral agents, before eventually switching to insulin. Several insulin regimens are suitable in type 2 diabetes and twice-daily injections of a premixed formulation (e.g. 30% short-acting and 70% isophane insulin) given with an insulin pen are convenient and effective in many patients. Combination of insulin with metformin or a sulphonylurea is of value in a few patients, particularly in those previously uncontrolled on a high dose of insulin (>60 U/day) alone.

Figure 12.13
Treatment schedule for type 2 diabetes. BMI, body mass index; FGB, fasting blood glucose; syndrome X, insulin-resistance syndrome (hypertension, abdominal obesity, dyslipidaemia).

Chapter 13
Diabetic ketoacidosis and hyperosmolar non-ketotic coma

Diabetic ketoacidosis is a state of severe, uncontrolled diabetes due to insulin deficiency, and characterised by high blood glucose and ketone body concentrations and acidosis. It requires treatment by insulin and intravenous fluids. Ketoacidosis is a serious condition with a mortality of 5–10% in Western countries, and is particularly dangerous in the elderly.

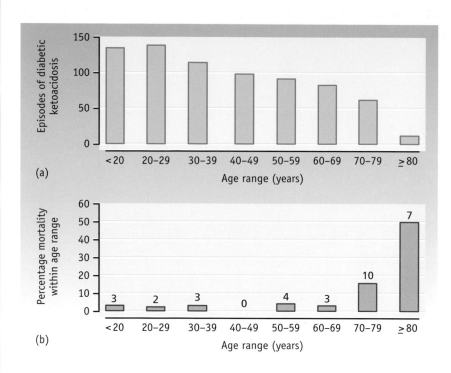

(a)

(b)

Figure 13.1
(a) Age distribution of 746 episodes of diabetic ketoacidosis (excluding paediatric cases). (b) Age distribution of deaths related to diabetic ketoacidosis ($n = 32$). Numbers of deaths in each age range are also shown.

The common precipitating causes of ketoacidosis are infection, management errors (especially giving the wrong dose of insulin or failing to increase dosage during intercurrent illness) and newly presenting type 1 diabetes. There is no obvious cause in about 40% of cases.

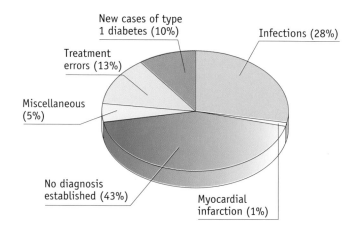

Figure 13.2
Precipitating causes of diabetic ketoacidosis.

Relative or absolute insulin deficiency in the presence of catabolic counter-regulatory 'stress' hormones (catecholamines, cortisol, glucagon and growth hormone) leads to hepatic overproduction of glucose and ketones. Insulin lack and stress hormones together promote lipolysis, with the release of non-esterified fatty acids from adipose tissue into the circulation. In the liver, fatty acids are partially oxidised to the ketone bodies, acetoacetic acid and 3-hydroxybutyric acid, which contribute to the acidosis, and acetone which is volatile and can often be smelled on the breath of ketoacidotic patients.

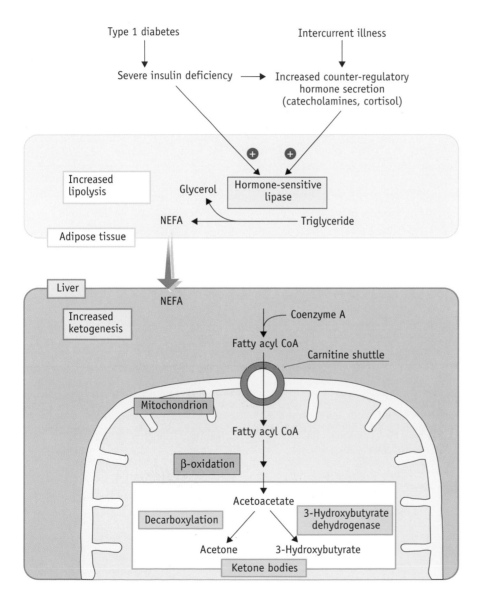

Figure 13.3
Mechanisms of ketoacidosis. NEFA, non-esterified fatty acids.

HANDBOOK OF DIABETES *2ND EDITION*

HANDBOOK OF DIABETES *2ND EDITION*

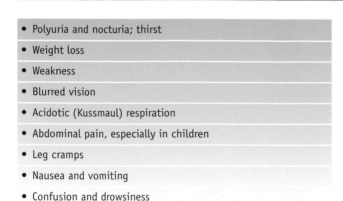

- Polyuria and nocturia; thirst
- Weight loss
- Weakness
- Blurred vision
- Acidotic (Kussmaul) respiration
- Abdominal pain, especially in children
- Leg cramps
- Nausea and vomiting
- Confusion and drowsiness
- Coma (10% of cases)

The symptoms of ketoacidosis include polyuria and thirst, weight loss, weakness, nausea, leg cramps, drowsiness and eventually coma (in about 10% of cases). Abdominal pain can occur, especially in younger patients. Signs include dehydration, hypotension, tachycardia, hyperventilation and hypothermia.

Figure 13.4
Clinical features of diabetic ketoacidosis.

Immediate bedside investigations should include blood glucose concentration and a test for the presence of urine or blood ketones (using a reagent strip), followed by laboratory tests, including blood glucose, Na$^+$, K$^+$ and bicarbonate, urea, arterial blood pH and gas tensions, and blood and urine culture.

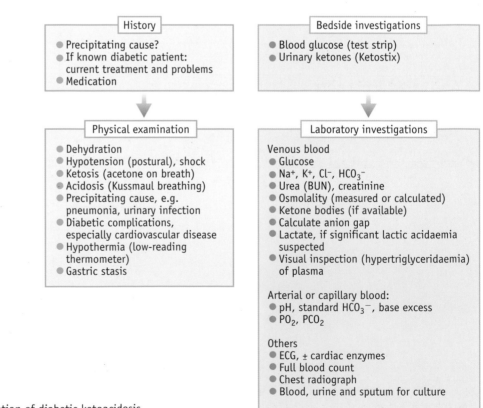

Figure 13.5
Flowchart for the investigation of diabetic ketoacidosis.

Fluids and electrolytes

Volumes

- 1 l/h × 3, thereafter adjusted according to need; usually 4–6 l in first 24 h

Fluids

- Isotonic saline ('normal'; 150 mmol/l)
- Hypotonic saline ('half-normal'; 75 mmol/l) if serum sodium exceeds 150 mmol/l (no more than 1–2 l—consider 5% dextrose with increased insulin if marked hypernatraemia)
- 5% dextrose 1 l 4–6 hourly when blood glucose has fallen to 15 mmol/l (severely dehydrated patients may require simultaneous saline infusion)
- Sodium bicarbonate (700 ml of 1.3% or 100 ml of 8.4% if large vein cannulated) if pH<7.0

Extra potassium should be given to prevent hypokalaemia

Potassium

- No potassium in first 1 l unless initial plasma potassium <3.5 mmol/l
- Thereafter, add dosages below to each 1 l of fluid:

  If plasma K⁺:

  <3.5 mmol/l, add 40 mmol KCl (severe hypokalaemia may require more aggressive KCl replacement)

  3.5–5.5 mmol/l, add 20 mmol KCl

  >5.5 mmol/l, add no KCl

Note: 20 mmol of KCl = 1.5 g

Insulin

Continuous intravenous infusion:

- 5–10 U/h (average 6 U/h) initially until blood glucose has fallen to <15 mmol/l. Thereafter, adjust rate (1–4 U/h usually) during dextrose infusion to maintain blood glucose 5–10 mmol/l until patient is eating again
- Intramuscular injections:
  20 U immediately, then 5–10 U/h until blood glucose has fallen to 10–15 mmol/l. Then change to 10 U 6-hourly subcutaneously until patient is eating again

Treatment involves rehydration and isotonic saline; short-acting insulin, ideally by low-dose intravenous infusion (e.g. 5–10 U/h until the blood glucose reaches 15 mmol/l, then 2–4 U/h); and potassium replacement, generally 20 mmol/l of saline. Bicarbonate administration to correct acidosis is controversial and it is not usually given unless the blood pH is <7.0 or cardiorespiratory collapse seems imminent (in which case, 700 ml of a 1.3% bicarbonate solution over 30–60 minutes is suggested).

Figure 13.6
Guide to initial treatment of diabetic ketoacidosis in adults.

Complications of diabetic ketoacidosis include cerebral oedema (children are particularly at risk, see Diabetes in children, p. 200), adult respiratory distress syndrome and thromboembolism.

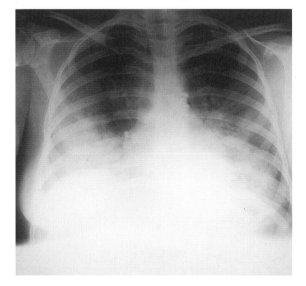

Figure 13.7
Adult respiratory distress syndrome. The chest radiograph shows typical bilateral shadowing, resembling that of pulmonary oedema due to left ventricular failure.

Hyperosmolar non-ketotic diabetic coma is characterised by marked hyperglycaemia (usually >50 mmol/l) and dehydration, without significant ketosis and acidosis. It usually occurs in middle-aged or elderly patients with type 2 diabetes, two-thirds of whom have previously undiagnosed diabetes. The absence of ketosis may be because of the residual endogenous insulin in type 2 diabetic patients, because hyperosmolality suppresses lipolysis or because counterregulatory hormone responses are less developed in these patients.

Hyperosmolar non-ketotic diabetic coma
• Marked hyperglycaemia
• Middle aged/elderly
• No ketosis/acidosis
• Often undiagnosed type 2 diabetes

Figure 13.8
Hyperosmolar non-ketotic diabetic coma.

Precipitating causes include infection, diuretic treatment and consumption of large quantities of glucose-rich drinks to quench thirst. Treatment comprises rehydration with isotonic saline, low-dose intravenous insulin infusion and potassium replacement, similar to the regimens used for ketoacidosis. After recovery, patients should be transferred to subcutaneous insulin injection therapy for a few months, but many can ultimately be controlled on diet alone or with an oral hypoglycaemic agent.

Chapter 14
Hypoglycaemia

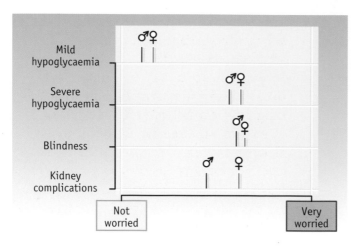

Figure 14.1
Attitudes towards different aspects of diabetes including severe hypoglycaemia, of 411 patients with type 1 diabetes, using visual analogue scales.

Hypoglycaemia is a common side-effect of treatment with insulin and some sulphonylureas. About 25–30% of insulin-treated diabetic subjects suffer one or more severe hypoglycaemic episodes every year (requiring assistance of others). It creates as much anxiety in insulin-treated diabetic patients as the long-term tissue complications, blindness and renal failure.

The main factors predisposing to moderate or severe hypoglycaemia include mismatch between the timing and/or amount of insulin and food, intensive insulin treatment, impaired awareness of hypoglycaemia, long duration of diabetes, exercise and excessive alcohol consumption. Counter-regulatory hormone deficiencies which increase insulin sensitivity, such as in Addison's disease and hypopituitarism, are rare.

Main causes of hypoglycaemia in diabetes

- Mismatch of food and insulin
- Strict blood glucose control
- Long duration of diabetes
- Hypoglycaemia unawareness
- Exercise
- Alcohol/other drugs

Figure 14.2
Main causes of hypoglycaemia in diabetes.

Autonomic	Neuroglycopenic	Malaise
Sweating	Confusion	Nausea
Pounding heart	Drowsiness	Headache
Shaking (tremor)	Speech difficulty	
Hunger	Incoordination	
	Atypical behaviour	
	Diplopia	

Figure 14.3
Common symptoms of acute hypoglycaemia in diabetic patients.

Hypoglycaemic symptoms can be classified as 'autonomic', due to activation of the sympathetic or parasympathetic nervous system (e.g. sweating, palpitations), or neuroglycopenic, due to the effects of glucose deprivation on the brain (e.g. drowsiness, confusion). Malaise is a non-specific symptom.

HANDBOOK OF DIABETES 2ND EDITION

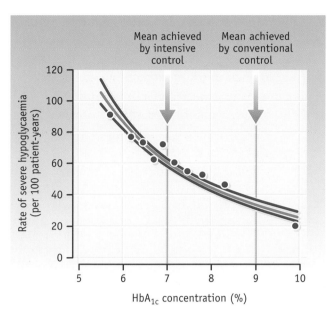

Figure 14.4
Relationship between the frequency of severe hypoglycaemia and the quality of glycaemic control, as measured by HbA$_{1c}$ in the DCCT trial.

The increase in the frequency of hypoglycaemia in well-controlled diabetes is seen particularly clearly in the Diabetes Control and Complications Trial (DCCT) where the rate of hypoglycaemia in the strictly controlled group of type 1 patients on an intensive insulin regimen (multiple insulin injections or CSII) was up to three times that in the conventionally treated patients. The two main reasons for this are thought to be lowering of the average glycaemic level which inevitably brings more troughs in blood glucose into the hypoglycaemic range, and the decreases in both the awareness of hypoglycaemia and the counter-regulatory hormonal responses to hypoglycaemia which occur with improved control.

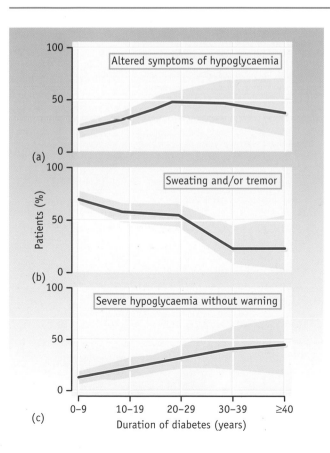

Hypoglycaemia unawareness increases with duration of diabetes, unrelated to glycaemic control; almost 50% of type 1 diabetic subjects with diabetes for more than 20 years have some degrees of unawareness.

Figure 14.5
Relationships between the duration of diabetes and the percentages of 411 diabetic patients reporting changes in symptoms of hypoglycaemia (a); sweating and/or tremor as one of their two cardinal symptoms of hypoglycaemia (b); and severe hypoglycaemia episodes without warning symptoms (c).

Unawareness may arise because patients with long duration of diabetes have a reduced counter-regulatory hormone response to hypoglycaemia. Glucagon is the first hormone affected and may be due to insensitivity of the islet A cell to hypoglycaemia; later, there is also a reduced catecholamine response to lowered blood glucose, both of which impair the blood glucose recovery from hypoglycaemia. Peripheral autonomic neuropathy is detectable in only some of the patients with hypoglycaemia unawareness, and probably plays a minor part in the causation.

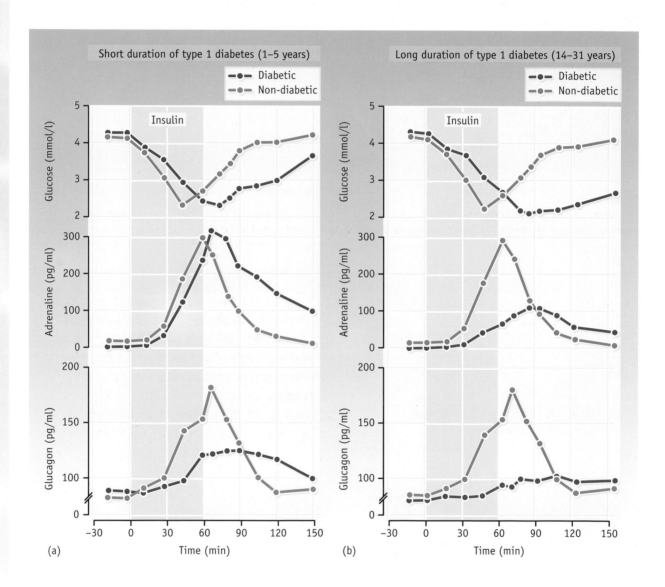

Figure 14.6
Impairment of counter-regulatory responses in type 1 diabetes: (a) after 1–5 years of type 1 diabetes, the mean glucagon response (lower panel) is blunted but the rise in adrenaline secretion is preserved (middle panel), glycaemic recovery is delayed (upper panel). (b) With long-standing type 1 diabetes, both glucagon and adrenaline responses are severely impaired and glycaemic recovery is markedly delayed and slowed.

HANDBOOK OF DIABETES *2ND EDITION*

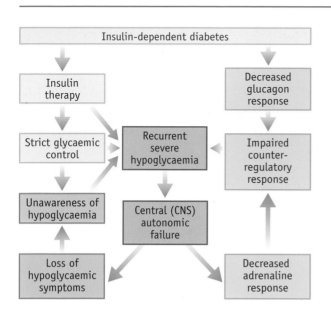

Counter-regulatory hormone deficiency and hypoglycaemia unawareness co-segregate and may have a common aetiology, possibly a defect in the recognition of hypoglycaemia by the central nervous system (central autonomic failure), caused by repeated exposure to hypoglycaemic episodes. This may also explain the unawareness associated with the institution of strict glycaemic control.

Figure 14.7
The hypothesis of hypoglycaemia-related central autonomic failure and its possible relationship to decreased symptomatic awareness of hypoglycaemia and to defects in the counter-regulatory hormonal responses.

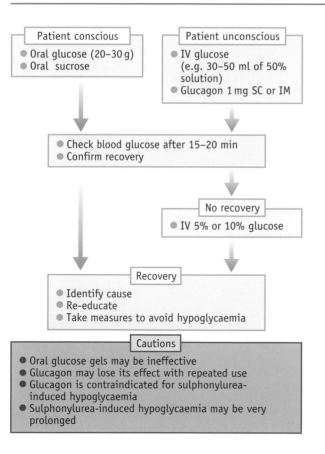

Suspected severe hypoglycaemia, e.g. in a diabetic patient with impaired consciousness or coma, must be confirmed by blood glucose testing (reagent strips). It should be treated immediately with oral glucose or, if the patient is unconscious or unable to swallow safely, with intravenous glucose or intramuscular or subcutaneous glucagon injection. Patients usually recover within minutes.

Figure 14.8
Algorithm for treating acute hypoglycaemia in diabetic patients. Some important cautions are also indicated.

Chapter 15
Control and complications

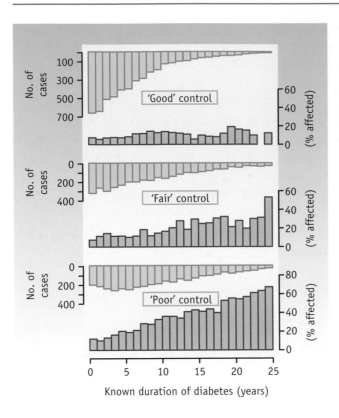

There is now strong evidence that the severity of microvascular complications in both type 1 and type 2 diabetes is associated with the duration and degree of hyperglycaemia. Diabetic patients with a lifetime of poor glycaemic control have a high frequency of tissue complications. A classical observational study by Pirart, which clearly demonstrated this link, followed some 4400 type 1 and 2 diabetic patients for up to 25 years; as the diabetes duration increased, the prevalence of retinopathy, nephropathy and neuropathy was highest in those with poor control and lowest in those with good control.

Figure 15.1
Prevalence of diabetic neuropathy as a function of duration of diabetes in patients with 'good', 'fair' and 'poor' control.

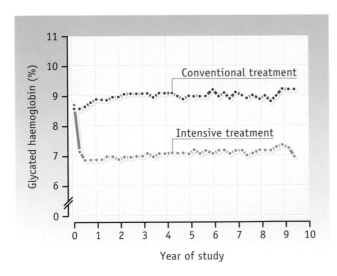

Figure 15.2
Glycaemic control achieved in the DCCT.

The definitive proof of the 'glucose hypothesis' for type 1 diabetes was the Diabetes Control and Complications Trial (DCCT, reported 1993). This large scale, prospective study is often regarded as a landmark in diabetes research. A total of 1440 patients at 29 centres in North America were randomly allocated to either conventional therapy (one or two daily insulin injections, 3 monthly clinic visits, no insulin dose adjustments according to self-monitoring data), or to intensive therapy (three or more daily insulin injections or CSII, monthly clinic visits and weekly telephone calls, frequent blood glucose self monitoring with dosage adjustment, diet and exercise programme). Throughout the 9- year study, there was a clear separation of glycaemic control in the two groups.

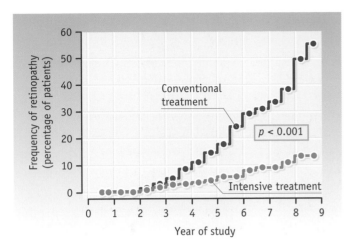

Figure 15.3
Effect of intensive treatment on the onset of retinopathy.
Cumulative incidence of background retinopathy in type 1
diabetic patients who entered the DCCT without retinopathy.

Clinically important retinopathy, nephropathy (urine albumin excretion) and neuropathy were reduced by about 35–75% in the group with strict control. For example, the cumulative frequency of retinopathy in those without this complication at the start of the study (primary prevention cohort) was reduced by an average of about 75% in the intensively treated patients. In those with initial early retinopathy (secondary prevention cohort), the average risk of progression was reduced by about 50%.

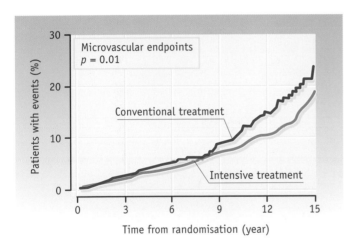

Figure 15.4
Effect of intensive blood glucose control on microvascular complications in type 2 diabetes (UKPDS).

Analogous evidence in type 2 diabetes for the role of strict glycaemic control in lowering the risk of tissue complications has come from the UK Prospective Diabetes Study (UKPDS, reported 1998). This 20-year study recruited over 5000 type 2 diabetic patients in 23 centres throughout the UK. In the main study, 3867 newly diagnosed type 2 diabetic patients were randomly allocated to either intensive therapy (the sulphonylureas chlorpropamide, glibenclamide or glipizide, or to insulin) or conventional therapy, which was diet initially, though tablets or insulin could be added later if symptoms or marked hyperglycaemia developed. Over 10 years, there was a reduction in HbA_{1c} from 7.9% with conventional treatment to 7.0% with intensive treatment, though in both groups glycaemic control deteriorated throughout the study. Intensive therapy in these type 2 diabetic subjects was associated with a significant 25% reduction in microvascular endpoints.

Both the DCCT and the UKPDS provide only borderline support for a reduction in macrovascular disease in diabetes by the institution of strict glycaemic control. It is generally believed that hyperglycaemia has a much less important role in the causation of macroangiopathy than it does in microangiopathy (see Macrovascular disease in diabetes, p. 153). Note however, that in a separate study within the UKPDS it was shown that a policy of tight blood pressure control in type 2 diabetes markedly reduced the risk of both micro- and macrovascular disease (see Hypertension in diabetes, p. 146), emphasising the 'bad companions' in diabetes of poor glucose and blood pressure control, to which one might also add dyslipidaemia and smoking.

Diabetes risk factors for complications

• Hyperglycaemia

• Hypertension

• Dyslipidaemia

• Smoking

Figure 15.5
Diabetes: the bad companions.

Glucose appears to damage tissues by acute reversible changes in metabolism (e.g. sorbitol accumulation, increased NADH/NAD$^+$ ratio, decreased myoinositiol, early glycation) and by cumulative, irreversible alterations in stable macromolecules (forming advanced glycation end-products). Genetic susceptibility and other accelerating factors such as hypertension and hyperlipidaemia also play a part.

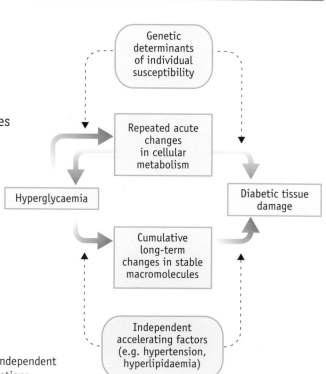

Figure 15.6
Scheme of the mechanisms by which hyperglycaemia and independent risk factors may interact to cause chronic diabetic complications.

HANDBOOK OF DIABETES *2ND EDITION*

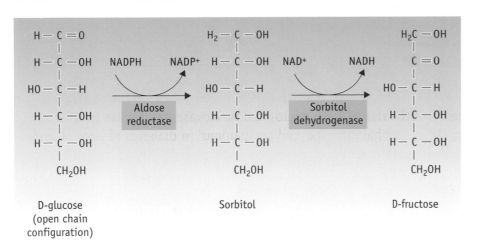

Figure 15.7
The polyol (sorbitol) pathway.

D-glucose (open chain configuration)

Sorbitol

D-fructose

Hyperglycaemia raises intracellular glucose levels in insulin-independent tissues such as nerve, glomerulus, lens and retina, where the enzyme aldose reductase catalyses the formation of the sugar alcohol, sorbitol, from glucose. In many tissues, sorbitol is subsequently oxidised to fructose using sorbitol dehydrogenase and NAD^+ as cofactor. Sorbitol does not easily cross cell membranes and accumulates intracellularly. It may cause damage through its osmotic effects (e.g. in the lens), by increasing the $NADH/NAD^+$ ratio ('pseudohypoxia') and by depleting intracellular myoinositol.

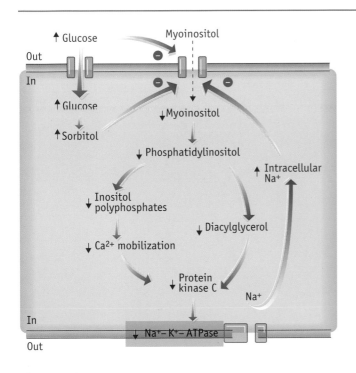

Figure 15.8
Possible mechanisms of intracellular myoinositol depletion under hyperglycaemic conditions, and the ways in which this could lead to impaired nerve function in diabetes.

Myoinositol is structurally related to glucose and mainly derived from the diet. Present in high concentrations in the cell, it is a precursor of phosphatidylinositol, which directly, or through mediators such as diacylglycerol, activates Na^+-K^+-ATPase in the neuronal membrane. Glucose and/or sorbitol may compete with myoinositol and block its uptake into cells. Diminished Na^+-K^+-ATPase activity leads to Na^+ accumulation in nerve cells, slowing nerve conduction velocity and further impeding myoinositol uptake.

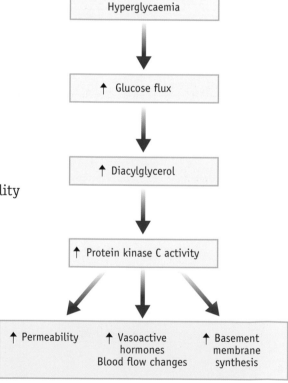

Several aldose reductase inhibitors have been undergoing clinical trials to test the effect of blocking the sorbitol pathway on the evolution of diabetic complications. Though there are encouraging results in some animal studies, the human trials are so far inconsistent.

Figure 15.9
Structures of the aldose reductase inhibitors, sorbinil (CP456634), ponalrestat (Statil) and tolrestat.

In other tissues, hyperglycaemia leads to *de novo* synthesis of diacylglycerol and activation of the enzyme protein kinase C. This enzyme has been implicated in several processes relevant to diabetic complications, such as increased capillary permeability and basement membrane synthesis.

Figure 15.10
Possible mechanisms by which increased *de novo* synthesis of diacylglycerol, causing stimulation of protein kinase C activity, could cause pathological effects in diabetic blood vessels.

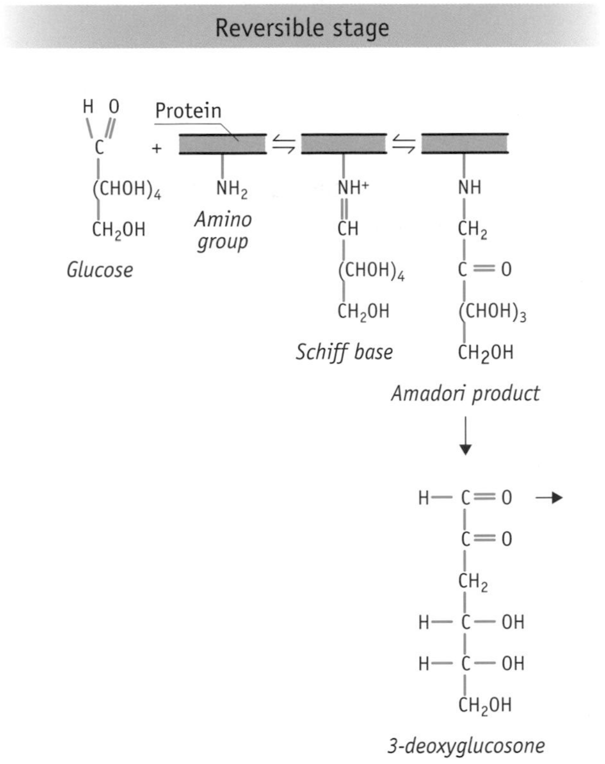

Reversible stage

Figure 15.11
Formation of reversible, early, non-enzymatic glycation products.

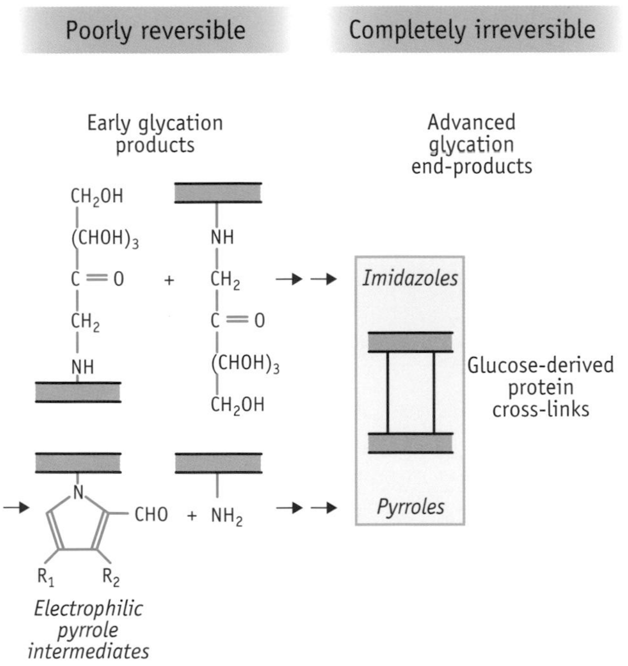

Glycation of proteins as the result of hyperglycaemia is initially analogous to the formation of glycated haemoglobin (HbA$_{1c}$), the widely used index of long-term glycaemic control. Glucose attaches non-enzymatically to amino groups on proteins, which then undergo a rearrangement to form more stable glycation (Amadori) products. Glycation may affect the properties of many proteins (e.g. the uptake of low-density lipoprotein into blood vessel walls is enhanced by glycation) and could be partly responsible for free radical-mediated tissue damage.

Poorly reversible　　**Completely irreversible**

Figure 15.12
Poorly reversible and completely irreversible glycation products. Through a complex series of chemical reactions, Amadori products can form families of imidazole- and pyrrole-based glucose-derived crosslinks.

With chronic hyperglycaemia, Amadori products in long-lived molecules like collagen and DNA combine to form cross-linked irreversible structures called advanced glycation end-products (AGE). The possible consequences of AGE formation include binding of low density lipoprotein (LDL) and other proteins by AGE-collagen in blood vessel walls, thereby predisposing to atherosclerosis, and disruption of structure and impaired enzymatic turnover of matrix proteins, leading to increased basement membrane permeability and thickening. AGE also bind to specific receptors on macrophages, kidney mesangial cells and endothelial cells, releasing prothrombotic cytokines and growth factors which cause cell proliferation.

As well as biochemical abnormalities, haemodynamic and haemorrheological disturbances accompany and sometimes precede microangiopathy, and may contribute to its pathogenesis. Early abnormalities include increased capillary blood flow and pressure, increased blood viscosity, red cell aggregation and hypersensitivity of platelets to aggregating agents. Increased pressure and flow could cause tangential shear forces on the endothelium, stimulating capillary basement membrane formation, and leading to hyperfiltration of fluid out of the capillary. Eventually, capillary thickening (sclerosis) limits vasodilatation, whilst rheological defects also cause impaired microvascular flow and tissue damage.

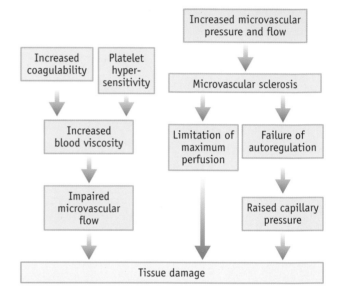

Figure 15.13
The 'haemodynamic hypothesis' for the development of diabetic microangiopathy.

Chapter 16

Diabetic eye disease

Diabetic eye disease primarily affects the retinal blood vessels, but diabetes also accelerates cataract formation (lens opacities). The lesions of diabetic retinopathy can be grouped into five categories, according to the features seen on ophthalmoscopy—background, preproliferative and proliferative retinopathy, advanced diabetic eye disease and maculopathy.

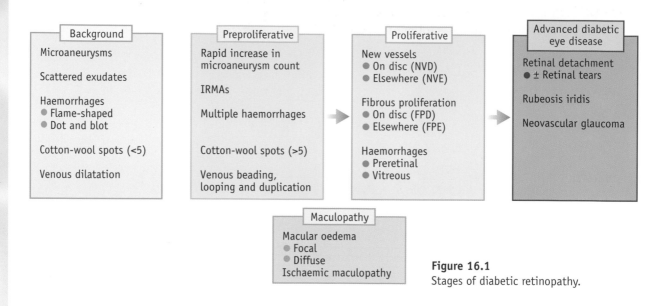

Background

Microaneurysms

Scattered exudates

Haemorrhages
- Flame-shaped
- Dot and blot

Cotton-wool spots (<5)

Venous dilatation

Preproliferative

Rapid increase in microaneurysm count

IRMAs

Multiple haemorrhages

Cotton-wool spots (>5)

Venous beading, looping and duplication

Proliferative

New vessels
- On disc (NVD)
- Elsewhere (NVE)

Fibrous proliferation
- On disc (FPD)
- Elsewhere (FPE)

Haemorrhages
- Preretinal
- Vitreous

Advanced diabetic eye disease

Retinal detachment
- ± Retinal tears

Rubeosis iridis

Neovascular glaucoma

Maculopathy

Macular oedema
- Focal
- Diffuse
Ischaemic maculopathy

Figure 16.1
Stages of diabetic retinopathy.

Background retinopathy is the first stage of retinopathy and is not associated with visual loss unless the macula becomes involved (maculopathy). Early sub-clinical abnormalities of the retinal vessels are basement membrane thickening, loss of pericytes (contractile cells which control vessel calibre and flow), and increased blood flow and capillary permeability. Microaneurysms are the earliest clinical sign of retinopathy (i.e. visible with an ophthalmoscope) and appear as red dots. They are blind out-pouchings of the capillaries, either at weakened points or a revascularisation response to microvascular occlusion.

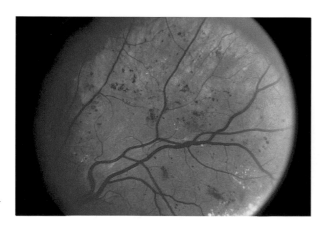

Figure 16.2
Background diabetic retinopathy, showing scattered red 'dots and blots' (microaneurysms and haemorrhages) and hard exudates.

Hard exudates are off-white/yellow flakes or plaques of plasma protein and lipid which have leaked from retinal blood vessels. They are most clinically significant in the area of the macula. Various forms of intraretinal haemorrhage also occur in background retinopathy (superficial flame-shaped, or deep 'dot and blot' and cluster haemorrhages). Cotton-wool spots are whitish elevations of the nerve fibre layer due to intracellular accumulation of axoplasmic material at areas of microvascular infarction.

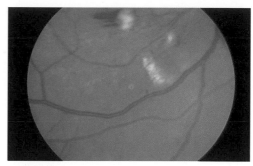

Figure 16.3
Cotton-wool spots with a nerve-fibre layer (flame) haemorrhage.

Preproliferative retinopathy is due to worsening retinal ischaemia and carries a high risk of developing into sight-threatening proliferative retinopathy. Early referral to a specialist ophthalmologist is required. Preproliferative changes include multiple cotton-wool spots (>5), multiple haemorrhages, venous 'beading' and intraretinal microvascular abnormalities (IRMAs, abnormally branched vessels in the retina, representing attempts to revascularise the ischaemic retina).

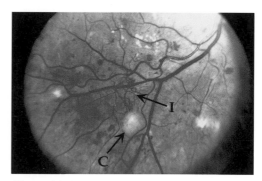

Figure 16.4
Proliferative retinopathy, showing cotton-wool spots (C), IRMA (I), and multiple, deep, round haemorrhages.

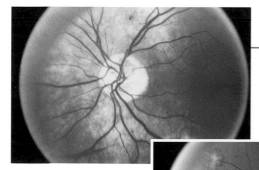

Figure 16.5
NVD. This photograph also shows a preretinal haemorrhage (at 7 o'clock).

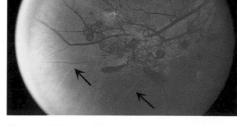

Figure 16.6
NVE, in this case below the macula of the right eye.

Proliferative retinopathy is marked by abnormal new vessels stimulated by growth factors released from the ischaemic retina. These new vessels grow forward towards the vitreous and overlie the retinal vessels. Contraction of the vitreous gel causes haemorrhage into the vitreous or the space between the gel and the retina. New vessels on the optic disk (NVD) are associated with the most severe retinal ischaemia and the worst visual prognosis, but neovascularisation also occurs elsewhere in the retina (NVE).

HANDBOOK OF DIABETES *2ND EDITION*

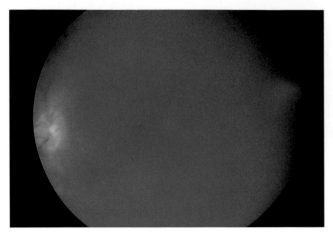

Figure 16.7
Preretinal haemorrhage.

Advanced diabetic eye disease comprises retinal detachment or tears, with preretinal (boat-shaped) or vitreous haemorrhages, which occur when further vitreous contraction pulls on strong fibrous adhesions connecting the retina and vitreous.

Sight can also be threatened by glaucoma due to neovascular tissue on the iris (rubeosis iridis) spreading peripherally on the pupil and obstructing the drainage of aqueous humour.

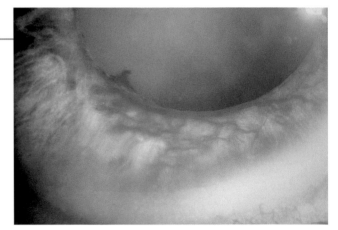

Figure 16.8
Iris neovascularisation (rubeosis iridis).

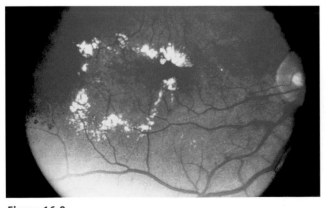

Figure 16.9
Maculopathy with circinate exudates.

Maculopathy is due to retinal oedema and thickening close to the macula, thus threatening or causing loss of central vision. Focal and diffuse maculopathy are caused by microvascular leakage, leading to fluid and hard exudates in the area of the macula. Ischaemic maculopathy is associated with areas of capillary non-perfusion and is difficult to detect. Hard exudates often occur in rings (circinate exudates) around the leaking area.

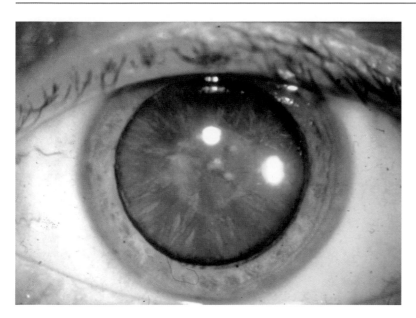

Figure 16.10
Diabetic cataract.

Cataract is a common cause of blindness in diabetic patients. It is recognised as an opacity against the red fundal reflex when the eye is examined with an ophthalmoscope at a distance of 30 cm. Non-enzymatic glycation of lens protein, especially α-crystallin, and subsequent cross-linking, probably contributes. Also, sorbitol accumulation in the diabetic lens could lead to osmotic swelling but the evidence for this mechanism in humans is less strong than in experimental diabetic cataracts in other species.

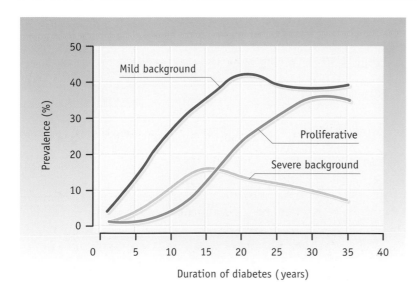

Figure 16.11
Prevalence of retinopathy (mild background, severe background and proliferative) according to duration of type 1 diabetes.

Diabetic retinopathy is the leading cause of blindness in the working population in the Western world. The prevalence of retinopathy increases with duration of diabetes, with few patients presenting with retinopathy in the first 5 years of diabetes and 80–100% developing some form of the complication after more than 20 years' duration. Maculopathy is most common in type 2 diabetes and can be associated with severe visual loss.

Figure 16.12
Indications for referring a diabetic patient to an ophthalmologist.

Condition	Urgency
Cataract	Routine (few months)
Retinal oedema/hard exudates: in the macula Retinal haemorrhages: numbers increasing Preproliferative changes	Soon (few weeks)
Fall in visual acuity (two lines or more) New vessels Rubeosis iridis Advanced diabetic eye disease, e.g. neovascular glaucoma	Urgent (1 week)
Retinal detachment Vitreous haemorrhage	Immediate (same or next day)

Regular examination of the eyes in diabetic patients for early detection of retinopathy is essential, and should include visual acuity measurement with a Snellen chart (uncorrected and corrected with spectacles or pinhole) and examination of the fundus through dilated pupils. When the retina cannot be seen because of cataract or haemorrhage, the patient should be referred to an ophthalmologist. Yearly examinations are recommended for those with no retinopathy, 6-monthly for those with background retinopathy, and referral to an ophthalmologist for cataract, maculopathy, increasing haemorrhages, proliferative and preproliferative changes, marked fall in acuity, retinal detachment, vitreous haemorrhage and rubeosis iridis.

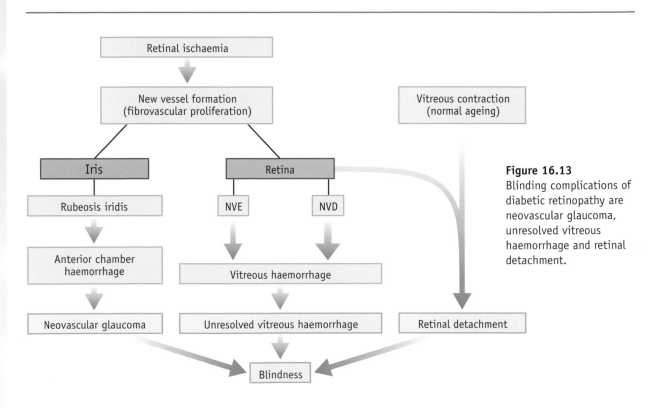

Figure 16.13
Blinding complications of diabetic retinopathy are neovascular glaucoma, unresolved vitreous haemorrhage and retinal detachment.

Blindness due to retinopathy can be caused by maculopathy, vitreous haemorrhage, retinal detachment and neovascular glaucoma, but visual loss can now be largely prevented by laser photocoagulation and vitreoretinal surgery.

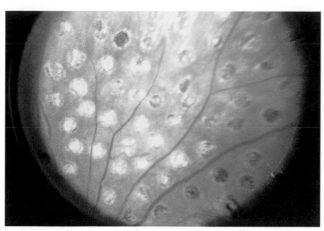

Figure 16.14
Panretinal photocoagulation. The whole retina is partially ablated apart from the macula and papillomacular bundle, to preserve central vision.

Panretinal photocoagulation, commonly with an argon (blue–green) laser, is used to treat new vessels and preproliferative retinopathy. The whole retina is partially ablated, except for the macula and papillomacular bundle which are essential for central vision. This concentrates the blood supply on the remaining retina and diminishes the ischaemic stimulus to new vessel formation. Established new vessels regress and further neovascularisation is inhibited.

Laser photocoagulation is also used to treat maculopathy; focal or grid (for diffuse or ischaemic maculopathy) treatment seals points of vascular leakage, reducing oedema and deposition of hard exudates. The 3-year risk of severe visual loss in maculopathy is reduced by over 50% with photocoagulation.

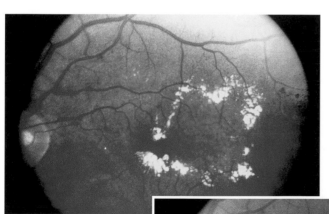

(a)

Figure 16.15
Focal photocoagulation for maculopathy: (a) before treatment; (b) one year later.

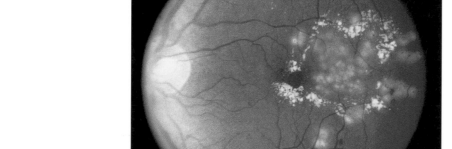

(b)

HANDBOOK OF DIABETES *2ND EDITION*

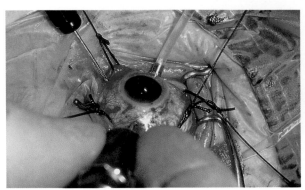

Figure 16.16
Vitrectomy, using common-gauge instruments inserted through the pars plana. Saline is infused through a cannula (top right) to maintain intraocular pressure; vitreous and contained haemorrhage is being disrupted with a cutter (bottom), illuminated by a fibre-optic light source (top left).

Closed vitreoretinal surgery employs microsurgery and endolaser photocoagulation to repair damaged retina, remove vitreous and haemorrhage and the membranes that cause retinal detachment. Tears in the retina can be repaired and reattachments made. This surgery can restore and maintain useful vision in up to 70% of eyes with advanced diabetic eye disease.

The results of the DCCT and UKPDS trials have shown the importance of both strict glycaemic and blood pressure control in reducing the risk of developing retinopathy. Recent evidence (e.g. the EUCLID study) also suggests that treatment of normotensive type 1 diabetic patients with an anti-hypertensive angiotensin-converting enzyme (ACE) inhibitor (lisinopril in the EUCLID study) markedly reduces the progression of established retinopathy and the incidence of new retinopathy.

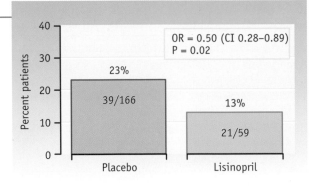

Figure 16.17
Progression of retinopathy by at least one level was halved (odds ratio 0.5) in type 1 diabetic patients treated with an ACE inhibitor (EUCLID study).

Whilst the value of ACE-inhibitor therapy in retinopathy needs to be further explored and is not yet established practice, medical treatments for retinopathy are likely to gain new importance in the coming years.

Chapter 17
Diabetic nephropathy

Figure 17.1
Photomicrographs showing glomerular basement-membrane thickening and mesangial expansion in the kidney of a diabetic patient. (a) ×1700; m, mesangial cell and matrix; us, urinary space; cap, capillary lumen. (b) ×4300, enlargement of boxed area in (a). EC, epithelial cell; G, glomerulus. Foot processes can be clearly seen.

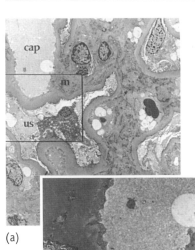

(a)

(b)

The main pathology in the diabetic kidney occurs in the glomerulus, where there is basement-membrane thickening within 2 years of diagnosis of diabetes and expansion of the mesangium (cells and matrix material which support the capillary tufts), eventually leading to a decrease in capillary filtering surface area and declining glomerular filtration rate (GFR). Nodular lesions which stain with periodic acid-Schiff (PAS) reagent on histological examination can occur in the central mesangium and when advanced give rise to nodular glomerulosclerosis or the 'Kimmelstiel–Wilson kidney'.

Proteinuria, detectable with a dip-stick (>0.5 g/day total protein) is usually the first manifestation of diabetic nephropathy and may be intermittent for several years. Once persistent proteinuria has developed, renal function usually declines gradually but progressively towards end-stage renal failure.

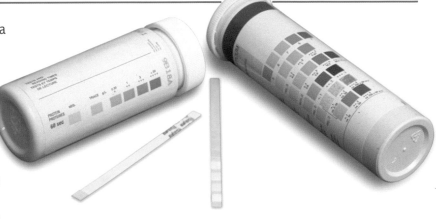

Figure 17.2
Dip-stick proteinuria detectable with reagent strips.

The natural history of diabetic nephropathy progresses from an initial stage of normoalbuminuria, through a phase of incipient nephropathy called microalbuminuria, where the increase in urinary albumin excretion can only be measured by sensitive immunoassay, to eventual dip-stick-positive proteinuria ('clinical' or overt proteinuria, or macroalbuminuria). Proteinuria thus increases as nephropathy progresses, though it only rarely reaches the proportions seen in the nephrotic syndrome. Progress may stop at any stage (occasionally regressing) and early death can occur, mainly from coronary heart disease (see Fig. 17.3).

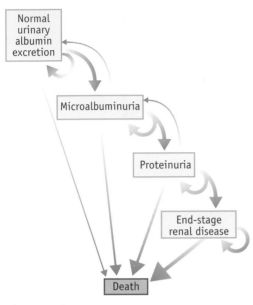

Figure 17.3
Natural history of diabetic nephropathy.

The prevalence of microalbuminuria, proteinuria and renal failure in diabetes increase with increase in duration of diabetes. About 30% of type 1 diabetic patients have proteinuria after 20 years' diabetes.

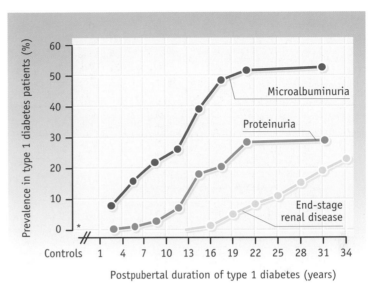

Figure 17.4
Prevalence of the stages of diabetic nephropathy according to postpubertal duration of type 1 diabetes.

Early microalbuminuria is due to an increase in transglomerular pressure, which is followed by loss of negative charge on the basement membrane and thus reduced charge repulsion between the membrane and the polyanionic albumin molecule. Macroalbuminuria supervenes when the pore size enlarges. With advanced renal failure, proteinuria becomes a mixture of glomerular and tubular defects, as the tubules' ability to reabsorb filtered protein is impaired.

Figure 17.5
Evolution of proteinuria in diabetes.
GBM, glomerular basement membrane.

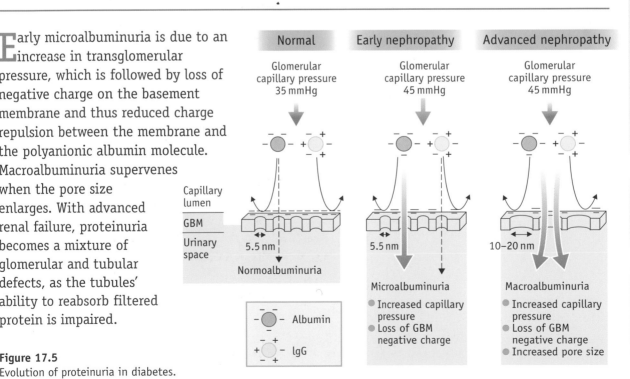

The urinary albumin excretion rate and thus the presence of microalbuminuria can be assessed by timed urine collections (e.g. microalbuminuria = 20–200 µg/min in an overnight sample or 30–300 mg/day). Because of problems of patient adherence, urinary albumin : creatinine ratio (ACR) in a random sample of urine is now a widely accepted measure in routine clinical practice.

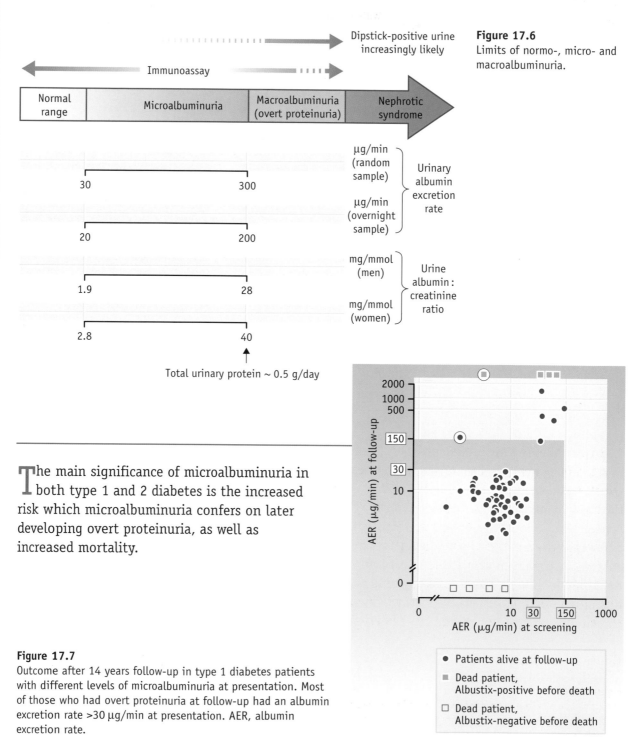

Figure 17.6
Limits of normo-, micro- and macroalbuminuria.

The main significance of microalbuminuria in both type 1 and 2 diabetes is the increased risk which microalbuminuria confers on later developing overt proteinuria, as well as increased mortality.

Figure 17.7
Outcome after 14 years follow-up in type 1 diabetes patients with different levels of microalbuminuria at presentation. Most of those who had overt proteinuria at follow-up had an albumin excretion rate >30 µg/min at presentation. AER, albumin excretion rate.

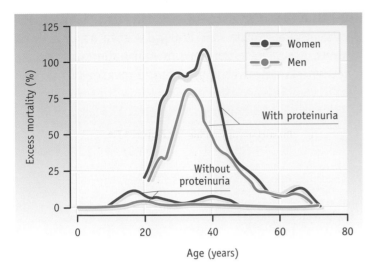

Proteinuria is associated with a high mortality, and indeed most of the excess mortality in diabetes is linked to proteinuria. About two-thirds of proteinuric diabetic patients develop renal failure and the rest die from cardiovascular disease.

Figure 17.8
Relative mortality of diabetic patients with and without persistent proteinuria in men and women as a function of age. Mortality is greatly increased at all ages in proteinuric patients.

Hypertension affects virtually all patients with persistent proteinuria. Diabetic nephropathy is also usually accompanied by widespread macrovascular disease, severe retinopathy, neuropathy and hyperlipidaemia.

The accompaniments to diabetic nephropathy
• Hypertension
• Macrovascular disease
• Severe retinopathy
• Neuropathy
• Hyperlipidaemia

Figure 17.9
Fellow travellers with to diabetic nephropathy.

Hyperglycaemia is clearly necessary for the development of diabetic renal damage, as shown by the DCCT and UKPDS trials of control and complications, but it is not sufficient. Other factors which may be involved include blood pressure and genetic predisposition. The incidence of retinopathy declines after about 15 years duration of diabetes, suggesting that there may be a subset of diabetic subjects who are especially susceptible to nephropathy. Familial clustering of nephropathy and hypertension suggest that some subjects may have a genetic propensity to nephropathy and/or hypertension. For example, the risk of developing overt nephropathy is increased threefold if at least one parent has hypertension.

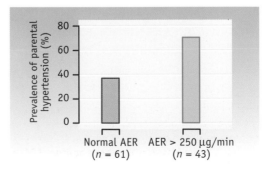

Figure 17.10
The prevalence of hypertension is increased in parents of those with proteinuria, suggesting that genetic predisposition may influence the development of nephropathy. AER, albumin excretion rate.

In those with microalbuminuria, normalisation of blood pressure, institution of optimal glycaemic control and correction of cardiovascular risk factors is recommended. Angiotensin-converting enzyme (ACE) inhibitors reduce urinary albumin excretion in non-hypertensive diabetic patients with microalbuminuria (*cf.* their effect in retinopathy and macroproteinuria). Although the long-term effect on renal failure is unclear, some physicians feel that these agents should now be used routinely at an early stage of nephropathy to slow the progression of the disease.

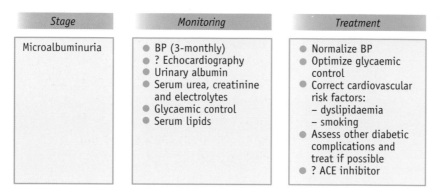

Figure 17.11
Management of microalbuminuria.

In those with overt proteinuria, renal function must be monitored to estimate prognosis and determine the effects of intervention. A 24-hour urine collection quantifies protein excretion, and urine should be examined microscopically and cultured to exclude infection. Ultrasound scanning can indicate renal artery stenosis. Serum creatinine does not increase until the GFR has fallen by 50–70%, so GFR should ideally be measured in the early stages by isotopic methods. Plots of inverse creatinine show a linear decline when the serum creatinine exceeds 200 μmol/l.

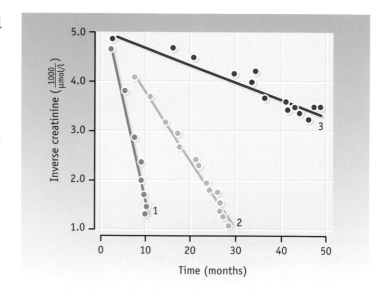

Figure 17.12
Inverse serum creatinine declines linearly with time, at a fixed rate for each individual patient (fastest for patient 1 and slowest for patient 3).

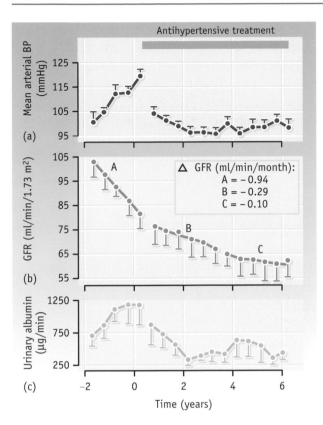

Figure 17.13

Effects of antihypertensive treatment on (a) mean arterial blood pressure; (b) GFR; and (c) urinary albumin excretion in type 1 diabetes patients with nephropathy. Rates of decline in GFR and albumin excretion were both significantly reduced.

Early, effective blood pressure control may delay the progression to end-stage renal failure. ACE inhibitors are generally thought to be the first-line agents for blood pressure control in diabetic nephropathy because they lower intraglomerular pressure as well as systemic blood pressure. Strict glycaemic control and moderate protein restriction are also indicated. As renal failure progresses, insulin requirements fall because of reduced renal clearance and degradation of insulin. Metformin and most sulphonylureas are also cleared by the kidneys and accumulate in uraemia causing hypoglycaemia and toxic effects. Transfer to insulin is therefore recommended when the serum creatinine exceeds 200 μmol/l.

Renal replacement therapy consists of haemodialysis, continuous ambulatory peritoneal dialysis (CAPD) and renal transplant. Renal transplant is the treatment of choice for those under 60 years and should be considered when the serum creatinine reaches about 500–800 μmol/l. Five-year survival exceeds 60% for cadaver grafts and 80% for live, related grafts at most centres.

Figure 17.14

Management of renal failure in diabetes.

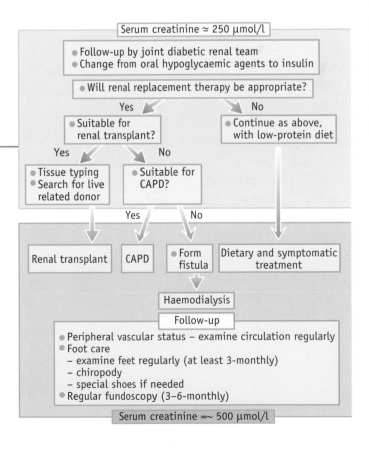

Patients with severe cardiac disease fare badly with renal transplantation and should probably be referred for dialysis. Gangrene and sepsis are further contraindications for transplant because of immunosuppression and the risk of infection.

| Age < 65 years |
| Absence of severe cardiovascular disease |
| Absence of severe cerebrovascular disease |
| Absence of significant sepsis |
| Suitable donor available |

Figure 17.15
Selection criteria for renal transplantation.

CAPD is inexpensive and suitable for elderly patients. No vascular access is required and because extracellular volume and blood pressure are stable it is suitable for those with heart disease or autonomic neuropathy. Good metabolic control can be obtained by adding short-acting insulin to the dialysis fluid.

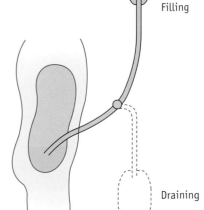

Figure 17.16
Continuous ambulatory peritoneal dialysis (CAPD). Dialysis fluid is instilled by gravity into the peritoneal cavity and drained after a dwell period of several hours.

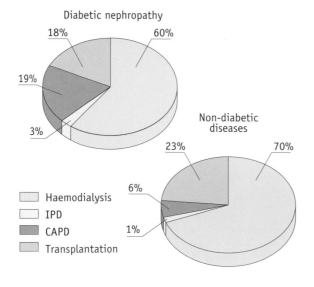

Chronic haemodialysis is the commonest form of therapy for end-stage renal failure in many countries, but it is complicated by difficult vascular access and failure of arteriovenous fistulae (which should be created 3–6 months in advance to allow for maturation), postural hypertension and erratic metabolic control.

Figure 17.17
Methods of renal replacement used to treat patients with diabetic nephropathy and other primary renal diseases throughout Europe. IPD and CAPD, intermittent and continuous ambulatory peritoneal dialysis respectively.

Chapter 18
Diabetic neuropathy

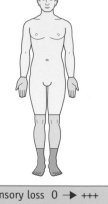

Symmetrical diffuse sensorimotor neuropathy

Sensory loss   0 ➡ +++
Pain   + ➡ +++
Tendon reflexes   N ➡ ↓
Motor deficit   0 ➡ +

There is no widely accepted classification of diabetic neuropathy, but a number of clinical syndromes are recognisable. The commonest neuropathy is distal symmetrical neuropathy, the 'classical' diabetic peripheral neuropathy. This is due to distal dying back of axons affecting the long nerves, and therefore the feet are often affected in a stocking distribution. Autonomic involvement is usual, though mostly symptomless.

Figure 18.1
Symmetrical diffuse sensorimotor neuropathy.

Symptoms in distal symmetrical neuropathy
• Asymptomatic
• Numbness

• Altered sensation
   – paraesthesiae
   – allodynia

• Pain

Distal symmetrical neuropathy may itself be symptomless but the feet are put at risk because of loss of pain sensation. Later, numbness and paraesthesiae and the feet feeling cold are characteristic symptoms. Pain (burning, or electric-shock like) and contact sensitivity (allodynia) can be extremely disagreeable. The hands are only rarely affected.

Figure 18.2
Symptoms in distal symmetrical neuropathy.

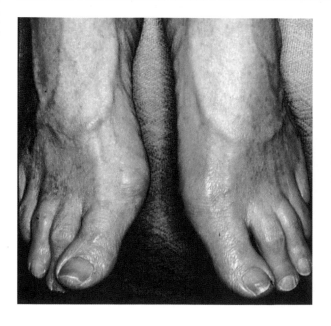

The most important complications are foot ulceration, neuropathic oedema (due to increased blood in the foot whose sympathetic innervation is damaged) and Charcot arthropathy (injury to the foot with reduced bone density because of increased blood flow causes chronic destruction, deformity and inflammation of the joints and bone—see The diabetic foot, p. 163).

Figure 18.3
Increased blood flow (distended veins) on the dorsum of the foot of a diabetic patient with painful peripheral neuropathy.

Signs in distal symmetrical neuropathy

- None

- Loss of vibration sense
  – pin prick
  – touch
  – temperature

- Wasting and weakness rare

- Complications (ulcer, oedema, Charcot arthropathy)

Examination may reveal distal symmetrical loss of vibration sense, pinprick and temperature. The clinical signs may be much less impressive than would be suggested by the patient's symptoms.

Figure 18.4
Signs in distal symmetrical neuropathy.

Diffuse small fibre neuropathy is a distinct syndrome, though a type of symmetrical distal neuropathy. It is characterised by loss of thermal and pain sensation (touch and vibration sense are intact) with symptomatic autonomic neuropathy (e.g. postural hypotension, abnormal sweating, diarrhoea), with increased blood flow to the feet, and frequently ulceration and Charcot arthropathy. Patients are often young, type 1 diabetic women. An autoimmune basis has been suggested.

Diffuse small fibre neuropathy

- Young, type 1 diabetes

- Often women

- Loss of thermal sensation

- Severe autonomic loss
  – postural hypotension
  – Charcot arthropathy
  – foot ulcers

Figure 18.5
Diffuse small-fibre neuropathy.

Figure 18.6
Femoral neuropathy.

Femoral neuropathy
(amyotrophy)

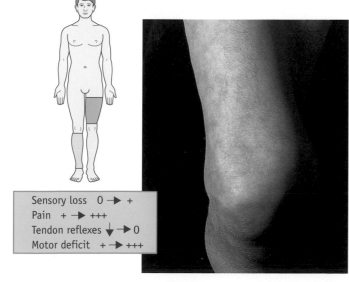

Sensory loss 0 → +
Pain + → +++
Tendon reflexes ↓ → 0
Motor deficit + → +++

In mononeuropathies, single nerves or their roots are affected. In contrast to distal symmetrical neuropathy, these conditions are of rapid onset and reversible, suggesting perhaps an acute vascular origin rather than chronic metabolic disturbance. The most well known is femoral neuropathy or diabetic amyotrophy. Typically, the patient is over 50 years of age, with continuous thigh pain, wasting and weakness of the quadriceps, and sometimes weight loss. Climbing stairs or getting out of a chair may be difficult. One or both thighs may be affected. Slow recovery, over many months, is usual.

Figure 18.7
Diabetic amyotrophy showing marked quadriceps wasting.

HANDBOOK OF DIABETES 2ND EDITION

Other mononeuropathies include cranial nerve palsies of the third or sixth nerves (causing diplopia). Truncal neuropathy causes localised bulging and neurogenic pain in the abdominal wall, either unilaterally or bilaterally. It is rare.

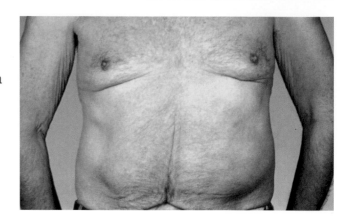

Figure 18.8
Bulging of the left lower abdominal wall due to truncal radiculopathy.

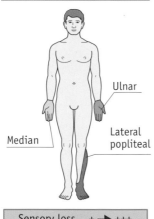

Pressure palsies occur because the peripheral nerves in diabetes are excessively prone to pressure damage. The commonest is carpal tunnel syndrome (median nerve palsy). Paraesthesiae and sometimes numbness occur in the fingers and hands. Discomfort can radiate into the forearm. Examination can show wasting and weakness of the thenar muscles, with loss of sensation over the lateral three and a half fingers. The diagnosis should be confirmed by nerve conduction studies. Most patients respond to surgical decompression.

Figure 18.9
Pressure palsies.

Ulnar nerve compression at the elbow causes numbness and weakness of the fourth and fifth fingers and wasting of the interossei muscles. Lateral popliteal nerve compression can cause footdrop.

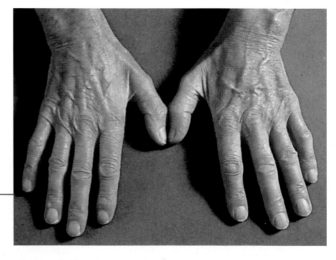

Figure 18.10
Generalised wasting of the interossei (and hypothenar eminence) due to bilateral ulnar nerve palsies in a diabetic patient.

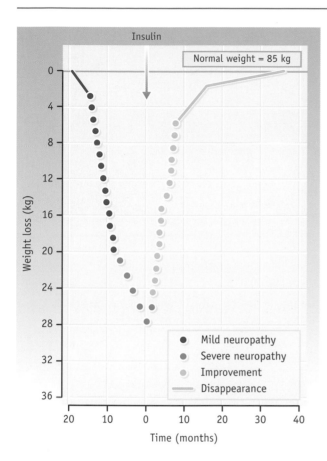

HANDBOOK OF DIABETES *2ND EDITION*

Acute painful neuropathy is frequently associated with marked weight loss. It sometimes develops 8–12 weeks after starting insulin treatment ('insulin neuritis').

Figure 18.11
Relationship between painful neuropathic symptoms and changes in body weight. Initiation of treatment with insulin is indicated by the arrow, treatment before then having been with an oral hypoglycaemic agent. A sudden loss of over 27 kg in weight is accompanied by the development of a mild and then a severe neuropathy. Restoration of body weight is associated with improvement and then disappearance of the neuropathy.

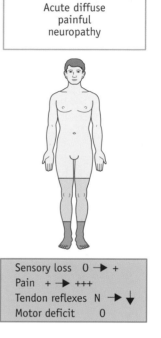

In patients with long-standing diabetes, numerous functional abnormalities can be demonstrated in organs receiving an autonomic innervation. Common manifestations are gustatory sweating (induced by eating) or other abnormal sweating, postural hypotension (systolic blood pressure fall >30 mmHg on standing), diarrhoea and impotence. Gastroparesis (delayed gastric emptying and vomiting) and bladder dysfunction are rarer.

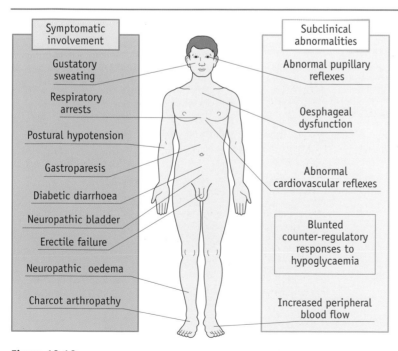

Figure 18.12
Clinical and subclinical features of diabetic autonomic neuropathy.

Both the DCCT and UKPDS trials of control and complications have confirmed that strict glycaemic control can decrease the risk of developing neuropathy, as judged by objective measures such as nerve conduction velocity. Attempts should be made therefore to optimise control. However, the main complaint of diabetic patients with neuropathy is pain, and there is as yet little evidence that improving control influences the intensity of neuropathic symptoms.

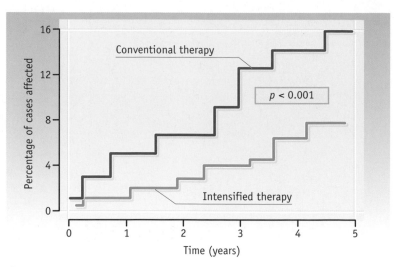

Figure 18.13
Effects of intensified insulin therapy and strict glycaemic control on the incidence of neuropathy in type 1 diabetic patients (DCCT).

Simple analgesics such as aspirin, paracetamol and codeine phosphate only rarely have an effect on diabetic neuropathic pain. Tricyclic antidepressants such as amitriptyline or imipramine, given at night, are most effective at controlling burning pain. Capsaicin (derived from hot peppers) is applied to the skin as a cream; it releases the peptide neurotransmitter, substance P, from pain-fibre nerve endings, leading to depletion of the nerves and insensitivity for several hours. Allodynia may respond to a bed cradle or a protective film (Opsite, Smith and Nephew) applied to the skin. Electric shock-like or 'shooting' pain may be treated with anticonvulsants (carbamazepine, phenytoin, valproate) or the orally active form of lignocaine, mexiletine. Restless legs are best managed by the benzodiazepine anticonvulsant, clonazepam. Cramps are generally helped by quinine sulphate at night.

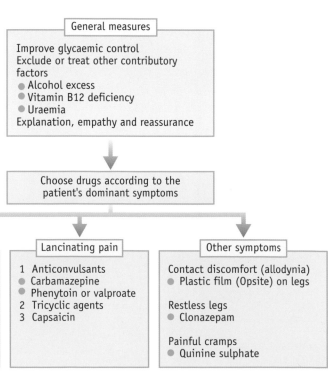

Figure 18.14
Approach to the management of painful diabetic neuropathy.

Chapter 19
Hyperlipidaemia in diabetes

Lipid abnormalities occur most commonly in diabetes in type 2 diabetic subjects, even in those who have reasonable glycaemic control. The characteristic pattern of blood lipids in type 2 diabetes is called 'diabetic dyslipidaemia' and consists of elevated serum total and VLDL (very low-density lipoprotein) triglyceride, low HDL (high-density lipoprotein) cholesterol and essentially normal total and LDL (low-density lipoprotein) cholesterol concentrations. The distribution of LDL subfractions, however, is altered, with a predomination of small dense LDL particles (sometimes called the 'type B' pattern) which are strongly related to vascular disease in the general population. Dyslipidaemia is also present in patients with impaired glucose tolerance.

Diabetic dyslipidaemia
↑ Triglyceride
↑ VLDL triglyceride
↑ Small dense LDL
↓ HDL-cholesterol

Figure 19.1
Diabetic dyslipidaemia.

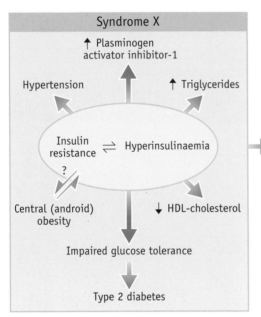

Figure 19.2
Insulin resistance syndrome (syndrome X).

Diabetic dyslipidaemia is a component of the insulin resistance syndrome (syndrome X), i.e. central or truncal obesity, hypertension, glucose intolerance, accelerated atherosclerosis, dyslipidaemia and insulin resistance.

Blood lipids in type 1 diabetes
Good control: 　No abnormality
Poor control: 　↑ cholesterol, ↑triglyceride, 　↑ VLDL, ↑chylomicrons, 　↓ HDL cholesterol

Figure 19.3
Blood lipids in type 1 diabetes.

In well-controlled type 1 diabetes, serum lipid and lipoprotein concentrations are similar to those in non-diabetic people. In poorly-controlled type 1 diabetes, there can be elevated levels of total cholesterol and triglyceride, very low-density lipoprotein (VLDL) and chylomicrons, and decreased high-density lipoprotein (HDL) cholesterol. The main determinants of hyperlipidaemia in type 1 diabetes are age, obesity, poor glycaemic control and nephropathy.

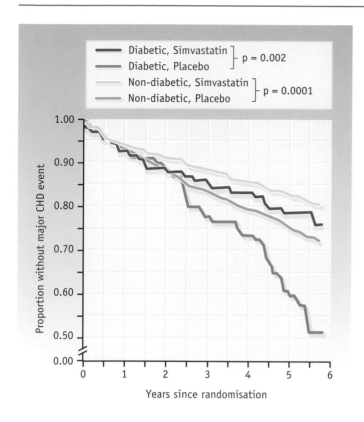

HANDBOOK OF DIABETES *2ND EDITION*

In type 2 diabetes, epidemiological studies have shown that serum triglyceride and lowered HDL cholesterol are more strongly associated with coronary heart disease than are total and LDL cholesterol. This may be because of the association of dyslipidaemia with the insulin resistance syndrome. There is little clinical trial information of the effect of lipid-lowering on coronary heart disease in diabetes, although a few trials have included a small number of type 2 patients. In the Scandinavian Simvastatin Survival Study ('4S'), simvastatin (a cholesterol-lowering drug—see p.141), reduced coronary heart disease incidence by 55% over 5 years in diabetic subjects with previously high LDL cholesterol and previous heart disease.

Figure 19.4
'4S' trial of the effect of simvastatin vs. placebo on CHD incidence in type 2 diabetes and non-diabetics.

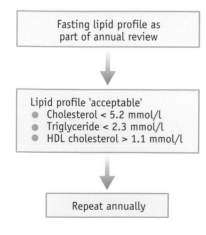

Total serum cholesterol and triglyceride and HDL cholesterol concentration should be routinely measured in diabetic patients, preferably on fasting blood samples. LDL cholesterol can be calculated (i.e. without direct measurement of LDL by ultracentrifugation) from the Friedewald formula (all concentrations in mmol/l, triglyceride should be less than 4.5 mmol/l)

$$LDL \; chol = [total \; chol] - [HDL \; chol] - \frac{[total \; triglyceride]}{2.2}$$

(note that this formula may be less accurate in diabetic subjects than normal subjects).

Figure 19.5
Routine lipid measurements.

Other medical disorders	Main lipid abnormalities
Alcohol abuse	↑ Triglyceride, ↑ HDL
Therapeutic drugs (diuretics, oral contraceptives, retinoids, corticosteroids, anabolic steroids, progestogens related to testosterone)	↑ Triglyceride and/or cholesterol, ↓ HDL
Hypothyroidism	↑ Cholesterol
Chronic renal failure	↑ Triglyceride
Nephrotic syndrome	↑ Cholesterol, ± ↑ triglyceride
Cholestasis	↑ Cholesterol
Bulimia	↑ Triglyceride
Anorexia nervosa	↑ Cholesterol
Pregnancy	↑ Triglyceride

Dyslipidaemias induced by antihypertensive drugs

	Total cholesterol	Total triglyceride	LDL cholesterol	HDL cholesterol
Calcium antagonists Vasodilators ACE inhibitors	N	N	N	N
Alpha-blockers	N↓	N↓	N↓	N↑
Diuretics	↑	↑	↑	N
Beta-blockers				
• Non-selective	N	↑	N	↓
• Intrinsic sympathomimetic activity	N	↑	N	N↑
• Vasodilator properties	N	N	N	N

Figure 19.6
Secondary hyperlipidaemia. N, no effect; ↑, ↓, reduced, increased levels.

Investigation of hyperlipidaemia in diabetes should exclude other secondary hyperlipidaemias, some of which are common in diabetes, such as hypothyroidism, drugs (e.g. alcohol, some antihypertensive agents), and renal disease. Primary hyperlipidaemia may also coexist with diabetes; severe hypertriglyceridaemia or cholesterolaemia in diabetic patients is often due to an underlying primary disorder, exacerbated by poorly controlled diabetes.

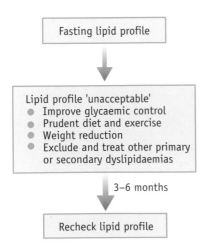

Figure 19.7
Treatment of hyperlipidaemia: initial measures.

Initial treatment of hyperlipidaemia in diabetes involves improving glycaemic control. This often produces an improved lipid profile in type 1 diabetes but may be insufficient to correct the dyslipidaemia of type 2 diabetes. Lifestyle measures should also be instituted, such as weight reduction in the obese, regular exercise and a low fat, lipid-lowering diet. Some replacement of carbohydrate with monounsaturated fats (e.g. olive oil) may be beneficial, especially in type 2 diabetes.

Figure 19.8
Modes of action of lipid-lowering drugs. Resins block the enterohepatic circulation of the bile acids by binding bile acids in the gut. This leads to increased bile acid synthesis and requirement for cholesterol in the liver. Nicotinic acid blocks lipolysis in the adipose tissue lowering NEFA and thus hepatic triglyceride and VLDL. Probucol blocks LDL oxidation and hence uptake by macrophages. Statins inhibit HMG-CoA reductase, reducing cellular cholesterol, up-regulating LDL receptor synthesis and LDL removal from the blood.

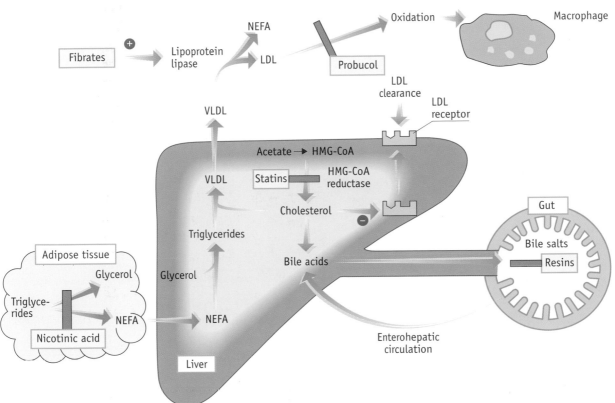

If hyperlipidaemia persists after these measures, lipid-lowering drugs should be considered. Statins (HMG-Co A reductase inhibitors, e.g. simvastatin, pravastatin, atorvastatin, fluvastatin, cerivastatin) are now the drugs of choice for lowering cholesterol. Statins inhibit an early step in cholesterol synthesis, which upregulates LDL receptor synthesis and promotes cholesterol removal from the blood. Fibric acid derivatives (bezafibrate, fenofibrate, gemfibrozil, ciprofibrate) are useful for hyperglyceridaemia and mixed hyperlipidaemia. They work partly by stimulating the enzyme lipoprotein lipase and the breakdown of triglyceride-rich lipoprotein. Other agents such as bile acid sequestrants, probucol and nicotinic acid derivatives are currently little used in diabetes.

Chapter 20
Hypertension in diabetes

WHO criteria for the general population	
Hypertension	Systolic > 165 mmHg Diastolic > 95 mmHg
Borderline hypertension	Systolic 140-165 mmHg Diastolic 90-95 mmHg

Hypertension-related tissue damage
  Grade I
  Grade II
  Grade III
	No damage
	Subclinical damage, proteinuria
	Clinical disease (or clinical damage)

Criteria for the diabetic population	
Hypertension requiring intervention	
Arbitrary threshold	Systolic > 140 mmHg
Above 95th centile of blood pressure for sex and old age	Diastolic > 90 mmHg

Figure 20.1
Definitions of hypertension.

Hypertension is as about twice as common in diabetes as in the non-diabetic population. Although the World Health Organization (WHO) defines hypertension as a blood pressure exceeding 160/95 mmHg, it is generally agreed that because of its many adverse consequences in diabetes, the threshold for defining hypertension should be lower in diabetes, say 140/90 mmHg. The British Diabetic Association has recently recommended a blood pressure of 140/80 mmHg or below as a treatment aim.

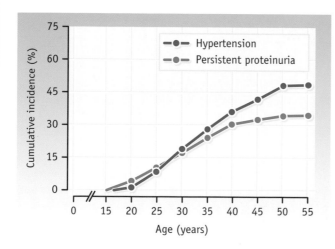

Figure 20.2
Cumulative incidence of hypertension and persistent proteinuria according to attained age in a cohort of juvenile-onset type 1 diabetes patients who were followed from the diagnosis of diabetes.

Using the WHO criteria, about 10–30% of patients of Caucasian type 1 diabetic patients have hypertension, the frequency closely related to the presence of nephropathy. Blood pressure usually starts to rise at the stage of microalbuminuria, and the incidence of hypertension parallels that of persistent proteinuria. This suggests that a genetic predisposition to hypertension might underlie the development of the renal complications in diabetes (see Diabetic nephropathy, p. 127). About 30–60% of white, type 2 diabetic patients have hypertension but there are marked differences in the frequency—there is low frequency in Mexican Americans and Pima Indians living in the USA.

In type 2 diabetes, hypertension is closely associated with metabolic syndrome X, or the insulin resistance syndrome (central obesity, hypertriglyceridaemia, low HDL cholesterol, accelerated atherosclerosis), with insulin resistance and/or hyperinsulinaemia being implicated as the common underlying factor. There are several ways in which increased insulin concentrations could lead to hypertension, including stimulating sodium and water reabsorption in the kidney; increasing intracellular sodium and calcium in the vascular smooth muscle which enhances contractility; causing hypertrophy of vascular smooth muscle; and stimulation of sympathetic nervous activity.

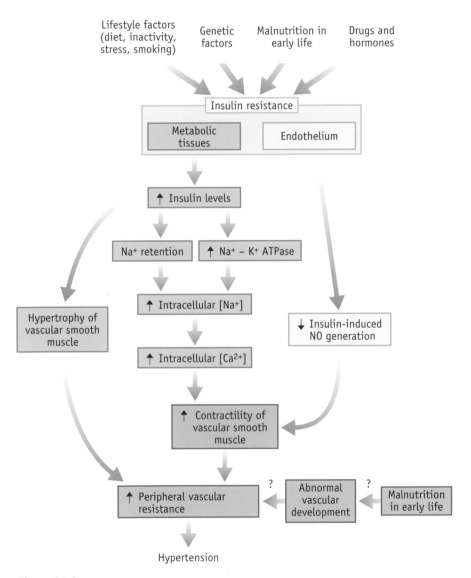

Figure 20.3
Possible basis of hypertension in patients with insulin resistance. Most of the effects are attributed to raised circulating insulin levels; resistance to the vasodilator effect of insulin—which is apparently mediated by release of nitric oxide (NO; also known as endothelium-derived relaxing factor [EDRF]) by the endothelium—may also contribute.

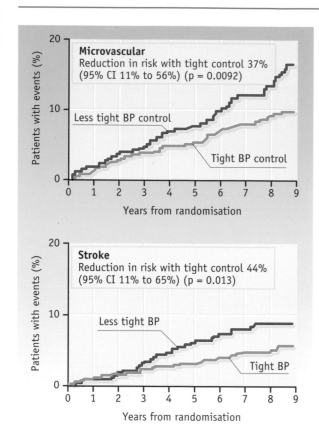

Figure 20.4
Kaplan–Meier plots of proportions of patients who developed microvascular endpoints (mostly retinal photocoagulation), and fatal and non-fatal strokes during tight or less tight BP control (UKPDS).

Control of hypertension in diabetes is important, not only because it is a major cardiovascular risk factor but because hypertension also accelerates microvascular complications such as nephropathy and retinopathy. This was clearly demonstrated in the recent UKPDS trial of control and complications (reported 1998), where 1148 hypertensive patients with type 2 diabetes were allocated to either tight control or less tight control of blood pressure (mean BP over 9 years 144/82 vs. 154/87 mmHg). Not only was there a large reduction in the risk of strokes (44%) but also of microvascular endpoints (37%), including retinopathy and microalbuminuria.

Initial investigations in hypertensive diabetic patients must exclude rare causes of secondary hypertension such as Cushing's and Conn's syndromes and phaeochromocytoma, and must assess renal damage (proteinuria or microalbuminuria, urine microscopy, serum urea, creatinine and electrolytes) and cardiovascular damage (ECG, chest X-ray for left ventricular hypertrophy). Other cardiovascular risk factors (hyperlipidaemia, poor glycaemic control, smoking, family history) should be identified.

Figure 20.5
Investigation of the diabetic patient with hypertension.

Investigations	Questions to be answered
History	Is hypertension significant?
Cardiovascular symptoms	Does hypertension have
Previous urinary disease	an underlying cause?
Smoking and alcohol use	• Renal
Medication	• Endocrine
Family history of hypertension	• Drug-induced
or cardiovascular disease	Has hypertension caused
	tissue damage?
Examination	• Left-ventricular
Blood pressure erect and supine	hypertrophy
Left-ventricular hypertrophy	• Ischaemic heart
Cardiac failure	disease
Peripheral pulses (including renal	• Cardiac failure
bruits and radio-femoral delay)	• Peripheral vascular
Fundal changes of hypertension	disease
Evidence of underlying endocrine	• Renal impairment
or renal disease	• Fundal changes
	Are other cardiovascular
Electrocardiogram	risk factors present?
Left-ventricular hypertrophy	• Smoking
Ischaemic changes	• Hyperlipidaemia
Rhythm	• Poor glycaemic control
	• Positive family history
Chest radiograph	of cardiovascular
Cardiac shadow size	disease
Left-ventricular failure	
Echocardiography	
Left-ventricular hypertrophy	
Dyskinesia related to ischaemia	
Blood tests	
Urea, creatinine, electrolytes	
Fasting lipids	

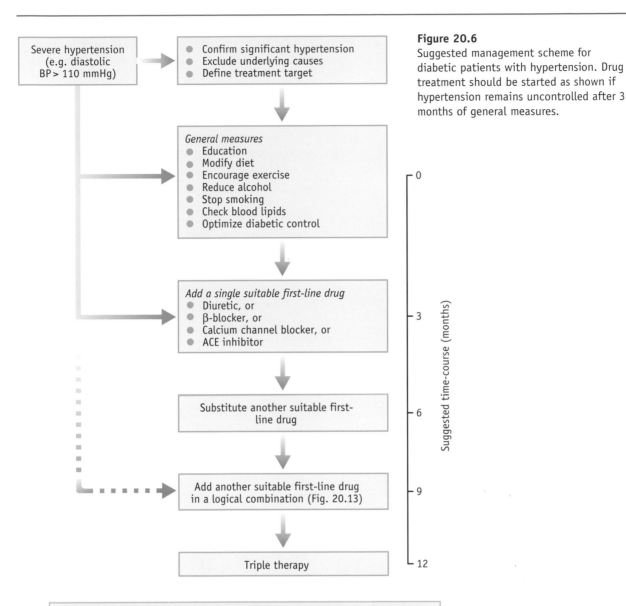

Figure 20.6
Suggested management scheme for diabetic patients with hypertension. Drug treatment should be started as shown if hypertension remains uncontrolled after 3 months of general measures.

Note: patients with severe hypertension will usually require single or double drug treatment from the outset; those with lesser degrees of hypertension frequently respond to general measures alone

Geneeral measures for the treatment of hypertension include weight reduction in the obese, low-fat/low sodium diet, increased physical exercise, institution of strict glycaemic control, reduced alcohol intake, cessation of smoking and management of hyperlipidaemia. These measures may be enough in those with mild hypertension to obviate the need for drug treatment. Patients with severe hypertension will generally need drug treatment from the outset.

HANDBOOK OF DIABETES *2ND EDITION*

First-line treatments for hypertension include ACE inhibitors (e.g. captopril, enalapril, lisinopril), diuretics (e.g. bendrofluazide), β-blockers (e.g. atenolol, metoprolol), and calcium-channel blockers (e.g. nifedipine, amlodipine, diltiazem, verapamil). There are a variety of relative indications and contraindications for each class of antihypertensive.

Group	Examples	Dosage	Relative indications	Relative contraindications	Precautions
Diuretics	Bendrofluazide Hydrochlorothiazide Indapamide Frusemide	1.25–2.5 mg o.d. 25 mg o.d. 2.5–5 mg o.d. 40–80 mg o.d.	Cardiac failure Renal failure (frusemide)	Hyperosmolar coma Impotence Gout Hyperlipidaemia	Give with potassium supplements or ACE inhibitors Monitor blood potassium Check blood glucose and lipids
Beta-blockers (cardio-selective)	Atenolol Metoprolol	50–100 mg o.d. 50–100 mg o.d.	Angina Previous myocardial infarction	Cardiac failure Heart block Peripheral vascular disease Impotence Asthma, chronic airflow obstruction Hyperlipidaemia	Warn about loss of hypoglycaemic awareness Monitor blood glucose and lipids
Calcium-channel blockers	Nifedipine Diltiazem Amlodipine	20 mg b.d. (sustained release) 90–240 mg b.d. 5–10 mg o.d.	Angina Arrhythmias	Significant cardiac failure Treatment with digoxin + β-blocker (verapamil)	Autonomic neuropathy (aggravate postural hypotension)
ACE inhibitors	Captopril Enalapril Lisinopril	12.5–50 mg b.d. (6.25 mg initially) 10–40 mg o.d. (2.5 mg initially) 10–40 mg o.d. (2.5 mg initially)	Cardiac failure Proteinuria	Renal artery stenosis Renal impairment	First-dose hypotension (use small starting dose at night) Monitor renal function Monitor plasma potassium (risk of hyperkalaemia)
Other agents	Doxazosin Hydralazine Clonidine	1–4 mg o.d. 25–50 mg b.d. 50–400 mg t.d.s.	Impotence Dyslipidaemia Renal failure Migraine		Use with diuretics and β-blockers First-dose hypotension

Figure 20.7
Antihypertensive drugs used in diabetes. First-line drugs are diuretics, β-blockers, calcium-channel blockers and ACE inhibitors. Dosage schedules; o.d., once daily; b.d., twice daily; t.d.s., thrice daily.

ACE inhibitors are popular first-line agents because they are not only effective in lowering systemic blood pressure but also delay the progression of diabetic retinopathy and reduce microalbuminuria, even in those without hypertension. They have no adverse effects on lipid profiles or glycaemic control, but they are less effective in lowering blood pressure in Afro-Caribbean patients. Dry cough (in 10–15% of patients) and potassium retention are recognised side-effects. Renal failure may occasionally be precipitated in those with renal artery stenosis. Exaggerated postural hypotension may occur with the first dose, especially in those overtreated with diuretics or with autonomic neuropathy, so that a low starting dose given at bedtime should be used.

ACE inhibitors

- Captopril
- Enalapril
- Lisinopril
- Perindopril
- Fosinopril
- Trandolapril
- Cilazapril

Figure 20.8
ACE inhibitors.

Angiotensin II receptor antagonists are a new group of anti-hypertensive drugs that block the action of angiotensin at its receptor. Losartan was the first to be introduced. At the moment, the clearest indication for these drugs is in patients in whom coughing has limited the use of ACE inhibitors.

Angiotensin II receptor antagonists
• Losartan
• Valsartan
• Irbesartan
• Candesartan

Figure 20.9
Angiotensin II receptor antagonists.

Calcium-channel blockers
• Nifedipine
• Amlodipine
• Diltiazem
• Verapamil

Figure 20.10
Calcium-channel blockers.

Calcium-channel blockers are vasodilators which normally have no adverse metabolic actions. Mild ankle oedema is a side-effect, and postural hypotension in those with autonomic neuropathy is exacerbated. Because of the vasodilator actions, they are useful in hypertensive patients with angina, but should not be used in those with heart failure because of an additional action of reduction in cardiac contractility—most potently with verapamil. The safety profile of the calcium-channel blockers is under review because of concern that they might increase the frequency of cardiovascular events, but the issue is currently unresolved.

A low dose of the thiazide diuretic, bendrofluazide (2.5 or even 1.25 mg/day), effectively lowers blood pressure in many patients; the risk of worsened glycaemic control and aggravated dyslipidaemia seen with thiazides is minimal at the low dose. Impotence and the precipitation of hyperosmolar non-ketotic coma are possible side-effects. If renal function is impaired, thiazides are without effect and loop diuretics such as frusemide are recommended.

Diuretics
• Bendrofluazide
• Hydrochlorothiazide
• Indapamide
• Frusemide

Figure 20.11
Diuretics.

Beta blockers
• Atenolol
• Metoprolol
• Propranolol
• Timolol
• Pindolol

Figure 20.12
Beta-blockers.

Beta-adrenoceptor blockers act mainly by reducing cardiac output. Atenolol and metoprolol are cardioselective. Propranolol and timolol are non-cardioselective and also act on bronchiolar smooth muscle to cause bronchospasm. They are contraindicated in patients with asthma. Like diuretics, they may aggravate hyperglycaemia, dyslipidaemia and impotence. Other problems with β-blockers are vivid dreams and cold hands and feet. β-blockers are, like ACE inhibitors, often less effective in Afro-Caribbean subjects.

Combination	Specific benefits	Disadvantages
Diuretics + ACE inhibitor	ACE inhibitor prevents activation of angiotensin–aldosterone system due to diuretic-induced ECF volume contraction, and helps to retain potassium	High risk of 'first-dose' hypotension with ACE inhibitor in patients overtreated with diuretics
Diuretic + β-blocker	—	Possibly aggravate hyperglycaemia in type 2 diabetes
Diuretic + calcium-channel blocker	Diuretic reduces mild ankle swelling due to calcium-channel blocker	—
Beta-blocker + calcium-channel blocker	Beta-blocker counteracts tachycardia due to calcium-channel blocker's vasodilator action Effective antianginal therapy	May aggravate or provoke cardiac failure (both are negative inotropes)

Figure 20.13
'Logical' double-drug antihypertensive therapy. ECF, extracellular fluid.

Treatment failures with first-line antihypertensives should be given, in sequence, an alternative first-line drug, then an additional first-line drug (certain combinations have proved safe and effective), and then either triple therapy or a second-line drug such as an α-receptor blocker (prazosin, doxazosin), or hydralazine.

Chapter 21

Macrovascular disease in diabetes

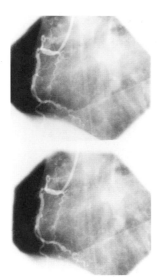

The frequency of coronary heart disease, stroke and peripheral vascular disease are all several-fold (about 2–4 times) higher in diabetic than non-diabetic subjects. Cardiovascular disease is the commonest cause of death in type 2 diabetes. Diabetic women are notably affected, since they lose the protection from cardiovascular disease enjoyed by non-diabetic women and have a relatively greater risk of atherosclerosis than diabetic men. Subjects with impaired glucose tolerance also have an increased frequency of cardiovascular disease.

Figure 21.1
Right coronary artery angiogram from a 50-year-old diabetic man, showing severe proximal and diffuse atheroma.

The pathology of atheromatous lesions in diabetes is identical to that in non-diabetic people, though the lesions may be more severe, extensive and run a more aggressive course. It is thought that injury to the endothelium by hyperglycaemia, hyperlipidaemia, smoking, etc. leads to monocyte and/or platelet adhesion. Monocytes migrate into the artery wall between the endothelial cells, become macrophages and accumulate lipid to form 'foam cells'. Release of growth factors and cytokines leads to migration and proliferation of smooth muscle cells which produce large amounts of connective tissue in the atherosclerotic plaque.

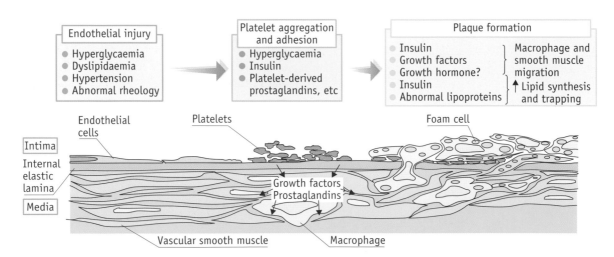

Figure 21.2
The pathogenesis of atheroma formation in diabetes. The initiating event seems to be injury to the endothelium of the artery, which may be caused by hyperglycaemia, dyslipidaemia or haemodynamic factors. Platelets aggregate and adhere to the exposed subintima and release platelet-derived growth factors and prostaglandins, which further encourage platelet aggregation. The growth factors, assisted by insulin and perhaps growth hormone, also stimulate the proliferation and migration of macrophages and vascular smooth muscle into the forming atherosclerotic plaque. Insulin stimulates lipid synthesis by the cells, which also take up abnormal LDL cholesterol via their 'scavenger' LDL receptors. The final atherosclerotic plaque consists largely of lipid-laden 'foam cells' derived from macrophages and vascular smooth-muscle cells.

The major cardiovascular risk factors in the non-diabetic population—smoking, hypertension and hyperlipidaemia—also operate in diabetes, but the risks are enhanced in the presence of diabetes.

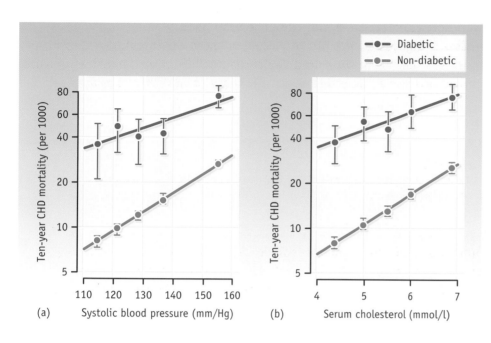

Figure 21.3
Effects of (a) systolic blood pressure and (b) serum cholesterol concentration on 10-year mortality from coronary heart disease (CHD) in 342 815 non-diabetic and 5163 diabetic subjects aged 35–57 years who had initially had not suffered myocardial infarction.

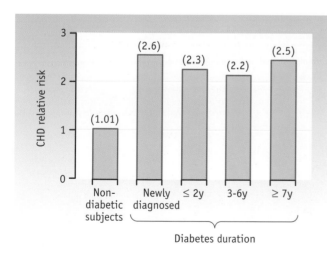

Figure 21.4
Relative risk of coronary heart disease (CHD) in type 2 diabetes is not related to the duration of diabetes.

This co-segregation of known risk factors only partially explains the cardiovascular risk of diabetes. The risk associated with diabetes itself is not fully explained. Unlike microvascular disease, there is a relatively weak relationship between macrovascular disease and either duration of diabetes or level of glycaemic control. This suggests that diabetes does not directly cause arterial disease but that another factor may predispose to both. One possibility for this 'diabetic' factor is hyperinsulinaemia and/or insulin resistance.

HANDBOOK OF DIABETES *2ND EDITION*

Many type 2 diabetic patients and most type 1 patients receiving conventional insulin injections have high circulating insulin concentrations. Animal studies indicate several possible mechanisms whereby insulin could promote atherogenesis, including stimulation of cholesterol synthesis in smooth muscle cells and macrophages of the arterial wall, stimulation of smooth muscle cell proliferation and migration, and enhancing the binding of LDL to smooth muscle cells and macrophages. Insulin can also raise blood pressure (stimulation of sympathetic nervous system, retention of sodium, increased smooth muscle contractility). Insulin also stimulates prothrombic processes such as the synthesis of VLDL and plasminogen activator inhibitor-1 (PAI-1, an inhibitor of fibrinolysis).

Changes in arterial wall

Increased cholesterol synthesis ⎤
Increased LDL binding   ⎦ Smooth-muscle and macrophages
Smooth-muscle hypertrophy and migration
Arterial wall thickening

Hypertension

Increased sympathetic nerve activity
Increased catecholamine release
Increased renal sodium retention
Increased Na⁺–K⁺ pump activity in smooth muscle (causes increased smooth
  muscle contractility)

Changes in blood

Increased VLDL synthesis in liver (increases triglycerides and LDL : HDL ratio)
Increased PAI-1 synthesis in liver, endothelium (inhibits fibrinolysis)

Figure 21.5
Possible atherogenic effects of insulin.

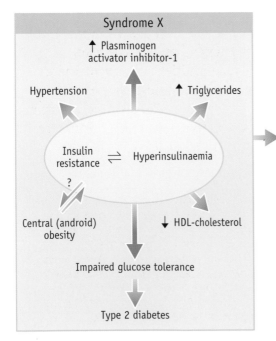

Figure 21.6
The 'insulin resistance syndrome' (syndrome X).

It is now well established that insulin resistance and hyperinsulinaemia are linked with a cluster of abnormalities called syndrome X, which include an increased risk of atherogenesis and coronary heart disease, impaired glucose intolerance or type 2 diabetes, dyslipidaemia, hypertension and truncal obesity. Other components of syndrome X include raised plasma uric acid and PAI-1 concentrations.

HANDBOOK OF DIABETES *2ND EDITION*

Microalbuminuria is a marker of cardiovascular risk in both diabetic and non-diabetic subjects. It may reflect not only increased glomerular capillary permeability but also more widespread endothelial damage, which could favour atherogenesis. Microalbuminuria, and the components of syndrome X may have their origin in genetically determined predisposing factors (insulin resistance, Na⁺/H⁺ pump activity) or reflect fetal or early neonatal malnutrition (the 'thrifty phenotype' hypothesis, see Epidemiology and aetiology of type 2 diabetes, p. 47).

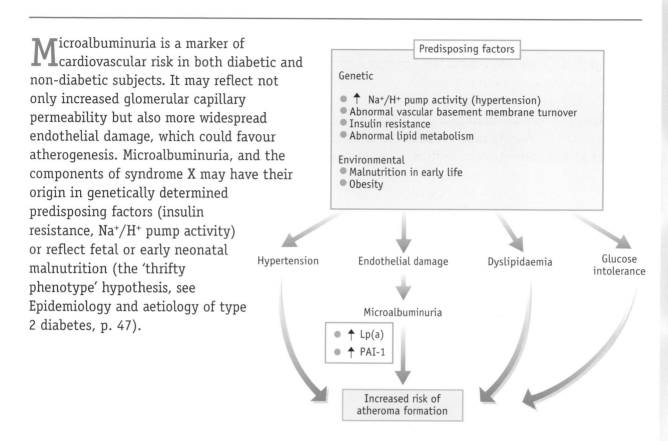

Figure 21.7
Possible links between microalbuminuria and cardiovascular risk factors in diabetes. Microalbuminuria is thought to reflect widespread endothelial damage.

Diabetes can also cause a cardiomyopathy, even in the absence of coronary artery atheroma. The main subclinical features are abnormalities of left ventricular contractility demonstrated on echocardiology, which generally correlate with duration of diabetes and extent of microvascular complications. More severe left ventricular dysfunction leads to heart failure.

Figure 21.8
Echocardiogram in a diabetic patient with severe congestive cardiac failure. (a) Long-axis, two-dimensional image in systole, showing dilated left atrium (51 mm) and left ventricle (55 mm). (b) Four-chamber, two-dimensional image in systole, showing biatrial and biventricular enlargement. There was global hypokinesia; dilation of the valve rings caused by functional mitral and tricuspid regurgitation, despite normal valves.

(a)

(b)

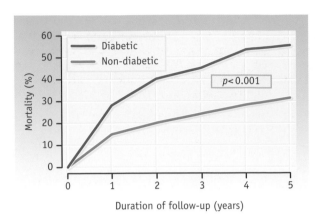

Figure 21.9
Five-year mortality among diabetic and non-diabetic patients during follow-up after myocardial infarction.

The presentation of ischaemic heart disease in diabetes involves angina, myocardial infarction and heart failure, as it does in the non-diabetic population. However, angina and myocardial infarction may be relatively painless in diabetes (perhaps due to neuropathic damage to the autonomic nerves serving the myocardium) and a presentation with just malaise, sweating, dyspnoea and syncope may be confused with hypoglycaemia. Both immediate and long-term mortality from myocardial infarction are increased in diabetes, largely due to the increased risk of heart failure in diabetes.

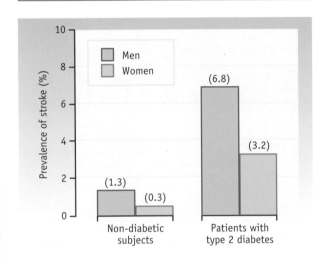

Mortality and disability from stroke are also worse in the diabetic person compared to non-diabetic people, perhaps because of the high blood glucose levels following the stroke. The presentation of a stroke in diabetes is similar to that in non-diabetic subjects, though the prevalence is increased.

Figure 21.10
Age-adjusted prevalence of previous stroke in type 2 diabetes subjects compared to control subjects (aged 45–64 years).

Arterial disease in the legs typically presents with intermittent claudication, i.e. calf pain on walking. Buttock pain may occur if the iliac vessels are affected and may be associated with erectile failure. Decreasing claudication distance and rest pain indicate critical ischaemia. People with diabetes have an approximately 16-fold higher risk of leg amputation than non-diabetic people (see The diabetic foot, p. 160).

Figure 21.11
Age-adjusted prevalence of intermittent claudication in type 2 diabetic subjects compared to control subjects (aged 45–64 years).

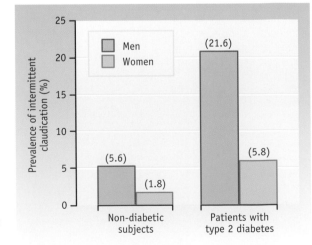

The management of myocardial infarction is similar to that in the non-diabetic population. Although there have been anxieties about the use of thrombolytic therapy in diabetes (e.g. streptokinase) because of the risk of promoting intraocular haemorrhage in the patient with retinopathy, therapy is highly effective in diabetes and intraocular bleeding is rare. Aspirin and β-blockers confer similar benefits in diabetic as in non-diabetic subjects in reducing reinfarction, and it is likely that ACE inhibitors, which reduce mortality, heart failure and reinfarction following myocardial infarction in non-diabetics, will also be effective in diabetes.

Management options after myocardial infarction in diabetic patients
• Thrombolytic therapy
• Aspirin
• β-blockers
• ACE inhibitors
• Tight glycaemic control
• Reduce risk factors

Figure 21.12

Management options after myocardial infarction in diabetic patients.

The use of a glucose–insulin infusion regimen to achieve tight glycaemic control after myocardial infarction may significantly reduce subsequent mortality.

Infusion mixture
Add 80 U soluble insulin to 500 ml 5% glucose Infuse initially at 30 ml/h Measure blood glucose every 1–2 h

Titrate infusion rate	
Blood glucose (mmol/l)	**Adjustment**
>15	Give 8 U soluble insulin as IV bolus Increase infusion rate by 6 ml/h
11–14.9	Increase infusion rate by 3 ml/h
7–10.9	Maintain current rate
4–6.9	Decrease infusion rate by 6 ml/h
<4	Stop infusion until glucose > 7 mmol/l Give 20 ml 30% glucose IV if symptomatic hypoglycaemia Restart infusion with rate decreased by 6 ml/h

Figure 21.13

Glucose–insulin infusion protocol to achieve tight glycaemic control following acute myocardial infarction.

HANDBOOK OF DIABETES 2ND EDITION

Efforts should be made to reduce cardiovascular risk factors in diabetic subjects, especially stopping smoking and treating hypertension. Recent small-scale trials show that there is benefit in reducing hyperglycaemia (e.g. the '4S' study, see Hyperlipidaemia in diabetes, p. 139). It is also sensible to aim for good glycaemic control, weight reduction in the obese and regular exercise, though the effects of these on cardiovascular disease in diabetes are less clear.

Reducing risk factors for cardiovascular disease
• Stop smoking
• Treat hypertension
• Treat hyperlipidaemia
• Improve glycaemic control
• Reduce weight in the obese

• Regular exercise

Figure 21.14
Reducing risk factors for cardiovascular disease.

Chapter 22
The diabetic foot

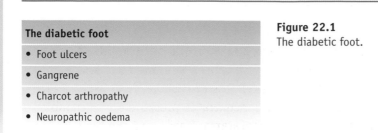

The diabetic foot

- Foot ulcers
- Gangrene
- Charcot arthropathy
- Neuropathic oedema

Figure 22.1
The diabetic foot.

Foot problems are a major component of diabetes care, the commonest lesions being foot ulcers, with or without infection, and gangrene. Charcot arthropathy and neuropathic oedema are rarer. The amputation rate amongst diabetic patients is over 15 times higher than in non-diabetic subjects.

The important causes of diabetic foot ulcers are neuropathy, and ischaemia due to macrovascular disease, but limited joint mobility, leading to abnormal foot pressures, and microvascular disease, impairing tissue nutrition and oxygenation, also contribute. Infection of ulcers probably occurs after the ulcer has been established, rather than causing it directly.

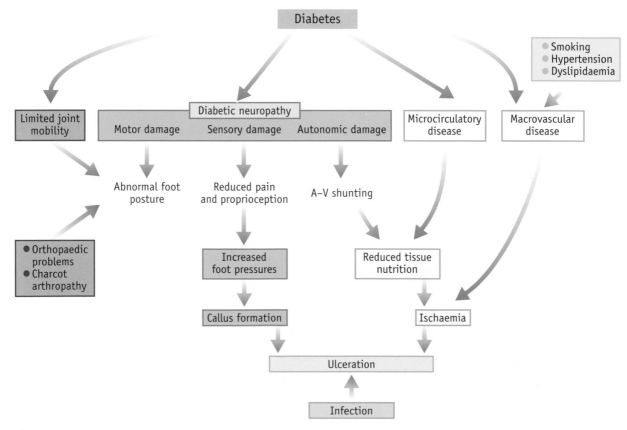

Figure 22.2
Pathways to foot ulceration in the diabetic patient.

Neuropathy predisposes to foot ulcers by reducing the perception of pain and discomfort with foreign bodies in the shoe, tightly fitting shoes and walking. Motor nerve damage causes weakness and wasting of the small muscles of the foot and, with loss of joint position sense, leads to altered posture of the foot. This concentrates pressure on vulnerable areas such as the metatarsal heads and the heel. Pressure stimulates callus formation, which is the precursor of ulceration.

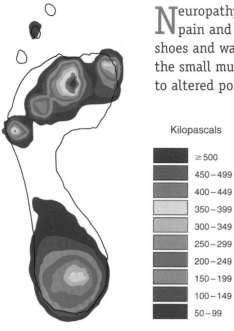

Kilopascals

▰	≥ 500
▰	450 – 499
▰	400 – 449
▰	350 – 399
▰	300 – 349
▰	250 – 299
▰	200 – 249
▰	150 – 199
▰	100 – 149
▰	50 – 99

Figure 22.3
Dynamic measurements of foot pressure under the sole, obtained during normal walking, using the optical pedobarograph. Pressure distribution, shown as contours.

Autonomic neuropathy plays a part by damaging sympathetic innervation of the foot, leading to arteriovenous shunting and distended veins. This bypasses the capillary bed in affected areas and may compromise nutrition and oxygen supply. Reduced sweating due to autonomic neuropathy leads to dry skin, which is prone to crack and provides a portal of entry for infection.

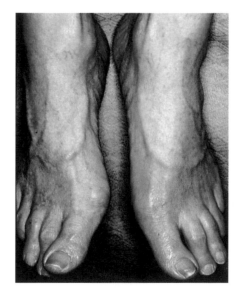

Figure 22.4
Distended veins on the dorsum of the foot of a diabetic patient with painful peripheral neuropathy.

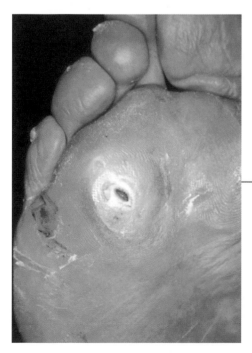

The typical neuropathic ulcer occurs on the plantar surface of the foot, or toes in high-pressure areas such as the metatarsal heads and heel, and has a 'punched-out' appearance, often with a surrounding callus.

Figure 22.5
Typical neuropathic ulcer. Note the surrounding callus.

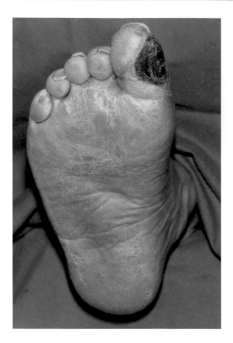

Ischaemia contributes to the formation of many diabetic foot ulcers. It usually acts in combination with neuropathy and infection. As well as major arterial occlusion, pre-existing microvascular disease probably contributes to the development of ulcers.

Figure 22.6
Neuroischaemic damage caused by tightly fitting shoes.

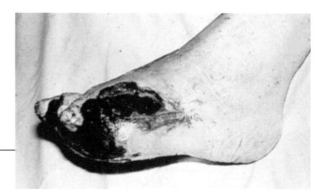

Figure 22.7
Gangrene localised to the forefoot in a neuroischaemic foot.

Predominantly ischaemic lesions, which are rare, result in gangrene that is localised to a specific area of the foot or to the entire foot in the worst cases.

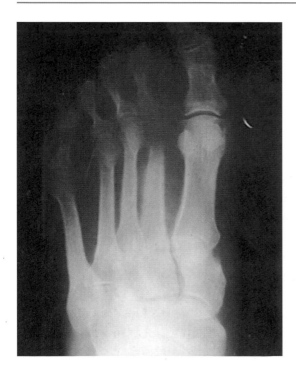

Infection of diabetic foot ulcers can be superficial or deep and potentially limb-threatening with abscesses and osteomyelitis. Systemic signs of infection such as fever are usually absent. Osteomyelitis should be assumed if bone can be felt on probing an ulcer. Plain radiography may reveal gas formation in the tissues, which indicates deep limb-threatening infection. Erosion of bone suggests osteomyelitis. ^{99m}Tc bone scanning and ^{111}In-labelled white-cell scanning can confirm osteomyelitis but differentiation from Charcot arthropathy and soft-tissue infection may be difficult.

Figure 22.8
Osteomyelitis. Bony destruction of the head of the second metatarsal visible on plain radiography, associated with a penetrating foot ulcer.

HANDBOOK OF DIABETES *2ND EDITION*

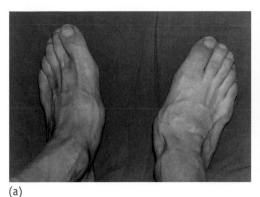

(a)

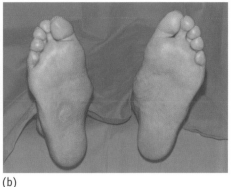

(b)

Figure 22.9
Bilateral Charcot neuroarthopathy in the cuneiform-metatarsal area that has resulted in characteristic deformity: (a) dorsal and (b) plantar views.

Charcot arthropathy occurs in patients with long-standing diabetes, and peripheral and autonomic neuropathy. The aetiology is poorly understood but it may be initiated by an injury causing a bone fracture. Increased blood flow may predispose by reducing bone density. Osteoclastic activity is stimulated but persists causing destruction, fragmentation, remodelling and gross deformity.

	Clinical examination	Objective testing
Shape and deformities	Toe deformities Prominent metatarsal heads Hallus valgus Charcot deformity Callus	Radiograph of foot Foot-pressure studies
Sensory function	Vibration (128-Hz fork) Thermal proprioception Semmes–Weinstein filaments	Biothesiometry Thermal-threshold testing
Motor function	Wasting, weakness Ankle reflexes	Electrophysiological tests
Autonomic function	Reduced sweating, callus, warm foot, distended dorsal foot veins	Quantitative sweat test Thermography for skin temperatures
Vascular status	Foot pulses, pallor, cold feet, oedema	Non-invasive Doppler studies, $TcPO_2$

Figure 22.10
Examination of the foot in diabetic patients.

Examination of the foot aims to assess the relative importance of neuropathic, ischaemic and infective components, as these require different treatments.

New approaches to wound healing undergoing trial

- Dermagraft
- Becaplermin gel
- Vivoderm autograft system

Figure 22.11
New approaches to wound healing undergoing trial.

Newer treatments for foot treatments for foot ulcers under evaluation include the topical application of products designed to accelerate wound healing. Dermagraft is a bioengineered human dermis consisting of neonatal fibroblasts cultured on a bioabsorbable mesh. It secretes matrix proteins and growth factors into the wound bed after implantation. Dermagraft is emerging as a new approach to the treatment of indolent plantar neuropathic ulcers which have failed to respond to conventional treatments. Becaplermin (Regranex) is a gel containing genetically engineered platelet-derived growth factor. It is used along with good wound healing practices to stimulate new tissue growth. Autologous cultured keratinocytes grown in a laser-perforated hyaluronic acid membrane (Vivoderm Autograft System) is also undergoing trial.

HANDBOOK OF DIABETES *2ND EDITION*

Target level of information to the needs and ability of the patient
Suggest 'dos' rather than 'don'ts' to encourage a positive approach

Do:
- Inspect feet daily
- Check shoes (inside and outside) before wearing them
- Have feet measured when buying shoes
- Buy lace-up shoes with plenty of room for toes
- Attend podiatrist regularly
- Keep feet away from heat (fires, radiators, hot water bottles) and check bath-water temperature before stepping in
- Wear protective footwear when indoors, or on the beach and avoid barefoot walking

Repeat the advice regularly

Also give advice to family members of the patient

Treatment and prevention of foot ulcers requires specialised assistance from the chiropodist (podiatrist) and shoe-fitter (orthotist), who should work closely with the diabetes team, and, when necessary, the orthopaedic and vascular surgeons. All patients must be educated about basic foot care and detection of abnormalities.

Figure 22.12
General principles of foot-care education.

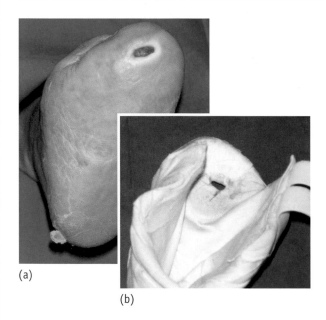

(a)

(b)

The key to management of neuropathic ulcers is relief of pressure, for example by encasing the foot in a light plaster-of-Paris cast, either with total contact or removable Scotchcast boot.

Figure 22.13
Neuropathic ulcer over the first and second metatarsal heads in a diabetic patient who (a) previously had the toes amputated for ulceration. (b) The foot was managed with a Scotchcast boot, with a hollow cut out under the ulcer area. Healing occurred within a few weeks.

Leg arteries should be investigated with non-invasive Doppler techniques and arteriography if appropriate. Severely affected patients, including those with localised gangrene, should undergo angioplasty or bypass surgery. Gangrenous toes should be amputated, and gangrene of the entire foot requires amputation, ideally below the knee.

Figure 22.14
Surgical approaches to ischaemic lesions of the diabetic foot. This patient presented with a gangrenous third toe; arteriography revealed extensive stenosis in the superficial femoral artery. A femoral–popliteal bypass was successfully performed, and the gangrenous toe amputated. Healing followed in a few weeks, and the patient was fully mobile soon afterwards.

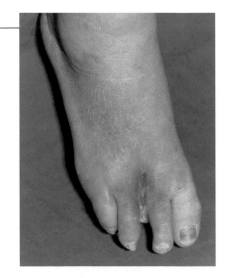

Chapter 23
Sexual problems in diabetes

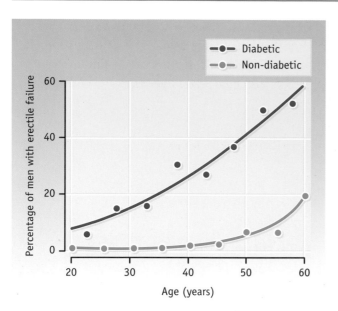

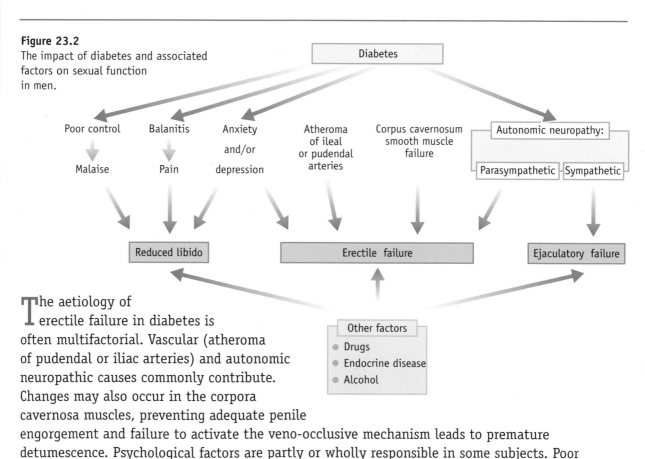

Erectile failure is the major sexual problem affecting diabetic men. It is very common, affecting up to 35% overall and about 60% of diabetic men over 60 years of age. Reduced libido and ejaculatory failure are other sexual problems which occur in diabetic men. The prevalence and impact of sexual problems in diabetes are probably underestimated because of social and medical taboos.

Figure 23.1
Prevalence of erectile failure in diabetic men.

Figure 23.2
The impact of diabetes and associated factors on sexual function in men.

The aetiology of erectile failure in diabetes is often multifactorial. Vascular (atheroma of pudendal or iliac arteries) and autonomic neuropathic causes commonly contribute. Changes may also occur in the corpora cavernosa muscles, preventing adequate penile engorgement and failure to activate the veno-occlusive mechanism leads to premature detumescence. Psychological factors are partly or wholly responsible in some subjects. Poor diabetic control can cause non-specific malaise and can be accompanied by lack of sexual interest. Balanitis, due to infection with *Candida*, is common in poorly controlled diabetes and can be sufficient to cause discomfort and anxiety, and to interfere with erection. Endocrine disease (e.g. testosterone deficiency, hyperprolactinaemia) is unusual.

Antihypertensive agents

β-adrenoceptor blockers
Thiazides and other diuretics
α-methyldopa

Antidysrhythmic drugs

Verapamil
Disopyramide
Flecainide
Propafenone

Lipid-lowering drugs

Fibrates

Psychotropic drugs

Antidepressants
Anxiolytics
Phenothiazines
Lithium

Miscellaneous

Allopurinol
Cimetidine
Ketoconazole
Metoclopramide
Non-steroidal anti-inflammatory agents

'Social' drugs

Alcohol
Smoking
Cannabis

Many drugs are associated with erectile failure, particularly alcohol, antihypertensive drugs such as β-blockers, thiazide diuretics and α-methyldopa, and antidepressants and anxiolytic agents.

Figure 23.3
Some drugs implicated in erectile failure.

History

What is the problem? (loss of libido, erectile failure, failure of ejaculation, penile problems)
What is its cause? (drugs, psychological, organic)
How important is it? (impact on patient and partner)
What needs to be done? (reassurance, active treatment)

Examination

Genitalia (balanitis, phimosis, Peyronie's, testes)
Cardiovascular system (leg pulses, iliac and femoral bruits)
Peripheral nervous system (neuropathy)

Routine tests

Testosterone
Sex hormone-binding globulin
Prolactin
Glycated Hb

Special investigations (not usually required)

Formal psychological assessment
Autonomic function tests
Nocturnal penile blood flow (Doppler)
Arteriography and cavernosography

Figure 23.4
Investigation of sexual dysfunction in diabetic men.

All diabetic men who complain of erectile failure or other sexual problems require a detailed history and examination. It is best to discuss and investigate these problems in a relaxed environment; the traditional busy diabetic clinic is usually unsuitable.

	More likely to be:	
	Psychological	Organic
Onset	Sudden	Gradual
Permanence	Intermittent or partial	Permanent and total
Spontaneous erections (nocturnal or on waking etc.)	Sometimes	Never
Psychological problems	May be overt	May be secondary
Organic causes	None apparent	May be apparent

Figure 23.5
Some factors that may help to differentiate psychological from organic causes of erectile failure.

It is important to distinguish between predominantly psychological and organic causes of impotence. Pointers towards a psychological basis include the persistence of spontaneous nocturnal erections, which normally occur during rapid-eye movement (REM) sleep or on waking; the ability to achieve erection on some occasions with the partner or when away from the partner; and the loss of erection after vaginal entry is attempted.

General measures

- Improve diabetic control
- Reduce alcohol intake
- Withdraw causative drugs
- Correct endocrine problems

Discussion and counselling (ideally with partner)

- Informal
- Formal sex or psychological therapy

Drugs

- Oral sildenafil
- Intraurethral alprostadil
- Intracorporeal vasoactive drugs (PGE, papaverine, phentolamine, VIP)
- Oral yohimbine

Vacuum tumescence devices

Surgery

- Correction of anatomical abnormalities (Peyronie's disease, phimosis, congenital, trauma)
- Implantation of penile prosthesis
- Arterial surgery (bypass or angioplasty)
- Correction of venous leakage

Treatment includes general measures to improve diabetic control, reduce alcohol intake, identify causative drugs and discussion and counselling. Recently introduced drug therapies include intraurethral prostaglandin (alprostadil, MUSE) and oral sildenafil (Viagra). In many cases, these are likely to supersede traditional treatments such as intracorporeal injection of vasoactive drugs, vacuum tumescence devices and surgical implantation of prostheses.

Figure 23.6
Treatment options for erectile failure.

Sildenafil is a selective phosphodiesterase inhibitor. Relaxation of the arterioles in the corpora cavernosa is mediated by nitric oxide release from nerve endings, which in turn increases intracellular cyclic guanosine monophosphate (cGMP); sildenafil inhibits the isoenzyme of phosphodiesterase which terminates the effect of cGMP, thus enhancing the erectile response to sexual stimulation. As sildenafil interacts with organic nitrates to cause acute hypotension, concurrent use with nitrates is contraindicated. Sildenafil is taken one hour before intended sexual activity (usually 50 mg, but 25 mg in older patients or those with renal or hepatic impairment). First experience of sildenafil in diabetes shows that it is effective in many patients (up to about 60%) and well tolerated.

Sildenafil (Viagra)

- Prevents cGMP breakdown
- Natural erectile response to sexual stimulation
- Probably effective in ~60% of diabetic patients
- Should not be given to those treated with nitrates

Figure 23.7
Sildenafil (Viagra).

Sexual problems in diabetic women

- Menstrual irregularities
- Infection
- Contraception
- Hormone replacement therapy
- Pregnancy

Figure 23.8
Sexual problems in diabetic women.

Common problems of sexual function in diabetic women relate to menstrual irregularities, infections, contraception, hormone replacement therapy and pregnancy. Menstrual abnormalities are common in diabetic women, particularly in those with obesity and poor glycaemic control. Insulin requirements alter around the time of menstruation in about 40% of diabetic women, mostly an increased need for insulin but about 10% needs less insulin.

Feature	Percentage of cases affected (range)
Menstrual abnormalities	
Amenorrhoea	25–50
Oligomenorrhoea	30–50
Regular cycles	15–25
Infertility	30–75
Masculinisation	
Acne	25
Hirsutism	60–70
Raised serum androgens	~80
Obesity	35–40
Glucose intolerance or type 2 diabetes	~40

Figure 23.9
Clinical features of PCOS.

Type 2 diabetes and impaired glucose tolerance are common in women with the polycystic ovary syndrome (PCOS)—features of which include oligomenorrhoea or amenorrhoea, polycystic ovaries on ultrasound examination, obesity, hirsuitism and raised circulating androgen levels. PCOS and type 2 diabetes/IGT share a strong association with insulin resistance. Possibly hyperinsulinaemia stimulates androgen synthesis and thecal hypertrophy in the ovary.

Genitourinary infections in diabetic women
• Vaginal candidiasis
• Vaginal warts, herpes
• Pelvic inflammatory disease
• Urinary tract infections

Figure 23.10
Genitourinary infections in diabetic women.

Genitourinary infections are common in diabetic women. Vaginal candidiasis is especially frequent in poorly controlled subjects; it can be very irritating and painful, and may interfere with sexual activity. Treatment involves improving control, and local or oral antifungal agents, including fluconazole. Genital herpes (HSV-2) and pelvic inflammatory disease in diabetic women may cause systemic upset, metabolic decompensation and ketoacidosis. Urinary tract infections are also frequent in patients with poorly controlled diabetes, and in those with autonomic neuropathy and bladder distension.

Combined oral contraceptive pills that contain low oestrogen doses are effective and have minimal metabolic side-effects in most cases. They are most suitable for young diabetic women without other cardiovascular risk factors (smoking, hypertension, hyperlipidaemia, positive family history). Combined pills that contain the progestogens desogestrel or gestodene may carry an increased risk of venous thrombosis and embolism and should be avoided if possible. For older women or those with diabetic complications or risk factors, progesterone-only pills are appropriate. These preparations are not thought to be associated with vascular disease. They may, however, cause menstrual disturbances, including intermenstrual bleeding and amenorrhoea.

Methods	Adverse effects on:		Thromboem-bolic risk	Other comments
	Glycaemia	Lipidaemia		
Combined — high-dose O + P, low-dose O + P, low-dose O + P, triphasic	+	+	+	Avoid combined pills if other risk factors for coronary disease are present: smoking, hypertension, hyperlipidaemia, positive family history
				Avoid pills containing desogestrel or gestodene (possible increased risk of thrombosis)
Progestogen only ('mini pill')	—	—	—	Menstrual irregularity. Use other contraceptive method if more than one pill missed (e.g. by omission, vomiting or diarrhoea).

Figure 23.11
Oral contraceptive pill and diabetic women. O, oestrogen; P, progestogen.

HANDBOOK OF DIABETES 2ND EDITION

Method	If method is used correctly	General outcome of method
Withdrawal	20	40
Rhythm method	10	25
Spermicides	10	20
Diaphragm	5	10
Condom	5	10
IUD	4	4
Contraceptive pill	<1	2
Vasectomy	<1	<1
Tubal sterilisation	<1	<1

Figure 23.12
The chances of pregnancy with various contraceptive methods: the number of women who will become pregnant for each 100 couples who used the method for 1 year is indicated. If no method is used, 80/100 women will become pregnant per year.

Intrauterine devices (IUDs) have no metabolic side-effects but may carry an increased risk of infection. There is some uncertainty about the suitability of IUDs in diabetic women but present evidence still supports the use of this contraceptive method. Condoms and diaphragms have a high failure rate, unless used carefully, but highly motivated couples may find these mechanical methods an effective and acceptable form of contraception, especially if combined with spermicidal cream or gel.

There has been reluctance to prescribe hormone replacement therapy (HRT) in postmenopausal diabetic women, possibly because of concerns about the risks of thromboembolism in the already procoagulant state of diabetes and the possibility of worsened glycaemic control. However, there is evidence that natural oestrogens and non-androgenic progestogens do not impair glycaemic control (they may increase insulin sensitivity and improve control) and improve lipid profiles (increase HDL, reduce LDL and PAI-1). It is accepted that HRT reduces mortality from coronary heart disease (CHD) in non-diabetic subjects. Because diabetic women are at increased risk of coronary heart disease, HRT should probably be more widely used. However, there are few if any long-term trials of HRT in diabetes.

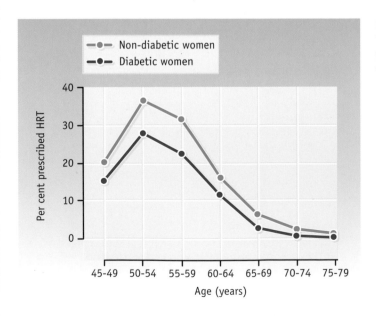

Figure 23.13
The percentage of women with diabetes who are prescribed HRT is less at each age group than in women without diabetes.

Chapter 24
Gastrointestinal problems in diabetes

Most gastrointestinal problems in diabetes relate to reduced motility due to autonomic neuropathy. Most patients have no or only mild symptoms, but a few can be disabled. The main clinical problems are associated with the oesophagus, stomach and bowel.

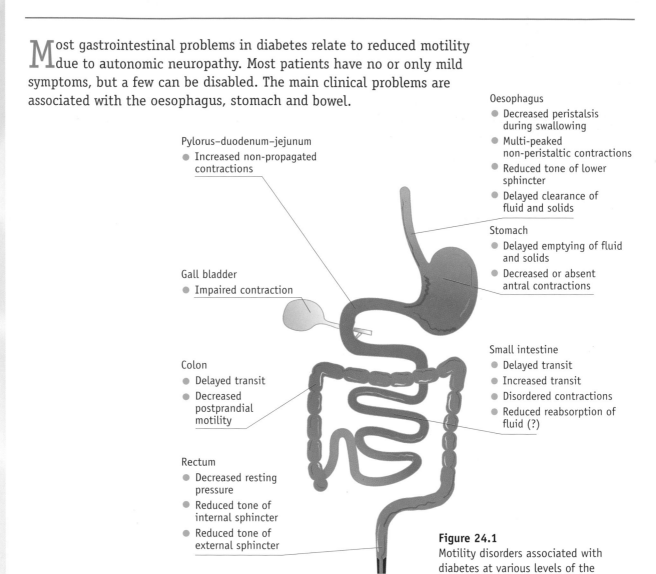

Pylorus–duodenum–jejunum
- Increased non-propagated contractions

Gall bladder
- Impaired contraction

Colon
- Delayed transit
- Decreased postprandial motility

Rectum
- Decreased resting pressure
- Reduced tone of internal sphincter
- Reduced tone of external sphincter

Oesophagus
- Decreased peristalsis during swallowing
- Multi-peaked non-peristaltic contractions
- Reduced tone of lower sphincter
- Delayed clearance of fluid and solids

Stomach
- Delayed emptying of fluid and solids
- Decreased or absent antral contractions

Small intestine
- Delayed transit
- Increased transit
- Disordered contractions
- Reduced reabsorption of fluid (?)

Figure 24.1
Motility disorders associated with diabetes at various levels of the gastrointestinal tract.

Symptoms of hypomotility of oesophagus and stomach
• Dysphagia
• Heartburn
• Epigastric fullness
• Anorexia
• Nausea and vomiting
• Weight loss
• Unpredictable glycaemic control

Figure 24.2
Symptoms of hypomotility of oesophagus and stomach.

Hypomotility of the oesophagus may cause dysphagia and acid reflux with heartburn. A barium swallow or endoscopy are required exclude achalasia, hiatus hernia, malignancy and monilial oesophagitis (which occasionally affects diabetic patients). Prokinetic drugs such as cisapride are useful for symptoms of dysphagia, though often less effective than in gastroparesis (see below). Heartburn responds to omeprazole or other proton pump inhibitors.

HANDBOOK OF DIABETES *2ND EDITION*

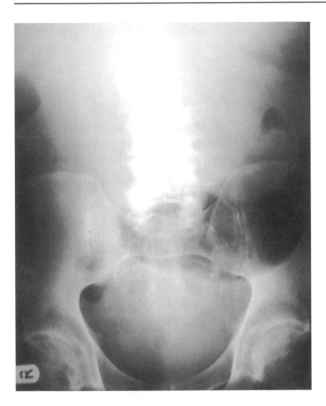

Gastroparesis, delayed emptying of the stomach, can cause anorexia, epigastric fullness, vomiting, chaotic glycaemic control and weight loss; it occurs with both autonomic neuropathy and in acute diabetic ketoacidosis. Examination can show epigastric distension and a succussion splash if the stomach is grossly dilated. A plain abdominal X-ray classically shows a 'ground glass' appearance in the upper abdomen.

Figure 24.3
Plain abdominal radiograph, showing uniform 'ground glass' appearance in the upper abdomen due to the greatly distended fluid-filled stomach of gastroparesis.

General measures
Maintain good glycaemic control. Eat small, frequent meals; avoid high-fibre foods
Oral prokinetic drugs • Cisapride • Metoclopramide • Domperidone • Erythromycin
Endoscopy indicated if
Haematemesis (usually due to Mallory–Weiss tear)
Other pathology or bezoar suspected
Severe episodes
Hospital admission
Intravenous rehydration
Intravenous prokinetic drugs • Metoclopramide 10 mg 4-hourly • Erythromycin 200 mg (3 mg/kg) 4-hourly
Nasogastric tube and drainage
Nutrition • Intravenous • Intrajejunal, via gastrostomy
Surgical drainage procedures as a last resort

Treatment of gastroparesis involves improving glycaemic control, eating small meals often and administration of prokinetic drugs such as cisapride (probably the drug of choice), domperidone, metoclopramide and erythromycin. Severely affected patients may need admission to hospital for intravenous fluid repletion, control of diabetes and possibly drainage of the stomach via a nasogastric tube. Endoscopy may be required to exclude other pathology.

Figure 24.4
Management of diabetic gastroparesis.

Diabetic diarrhoea

- Usually long-standing, poorly controlled diabetes
- Other evidence of autonomic neuropathy
- Diarrhoea often intermittent
- Diarrhoea often nocturnal

Figure 24.5
Diabetic diarrhoea.

Autonomic denervation and colonisation of the hypomotile bowel by colonic bacteria contributes to 'diabetic diarrhoea', but the aetiology is probably multifactorial. Diarrhoea is classically intermittent and often worse at night. Bouts lasting several days may be followed by spontaneous remissions. The diagnosis is by exclusion, and other possible causes of diarrhoea such as chronic pancreatic disease and coeliac disease must be eliminated.

Treatment of diabetic diarrhoea is by opioids (e.g. loperamide), or a broad-spectrum antibiotic such as tetracycline or erythromycin if bacterial overgrowth is proven or suspected. Troublesome diarrhoea, especially when watery, may respond to the α-adrenergic agonists clonidine or limidine. The long-acting somatostatin analogue, octreotide, may be helpful when other measures have failed.

Agent	Dosage
Opioid derivatives	
Codeine phosphate	30 mg, three to four times daily
Diphenoxylate hydrochloride	5 mg, four times daily
Loperamide hydrochloride	2 mg, three to four times daily
Broad-spectrum antibiotics (for bacterial overgrowth)	
Oxytetracycline	250 mg, four times daily ⎤ for 5–7 days
Erythromycin	250 mg, four times daily ⎦
Alpha-2-adrenergic agent	
Clonidine	0.3–0.6 mg, twice daily
Somatostatin analogue	
Octreotide	50–100 μg subcutaneously, two to three times daily

Figure 24.6
Drug treatments for diabetic diarrhoea.

Diabetic constipation

- Common (up to ~80% of those with neuropathy)
- Usually mild
- Tends to be neglected

Figure 24.7
Diabetic constipation.

Constipation is also common in diabetic patients with autonomic neuropathy, though it is usually mild. Other serious pathology such as colonic carcinoma must be excluded by rectal examination, proctosigmoidoscopy, colonoscopy or barium enema. If constipation requires treatment, stimulant laxatives such as senna or prokinetic drugs are usually effective.

Chapter 25
The skin in diabetes

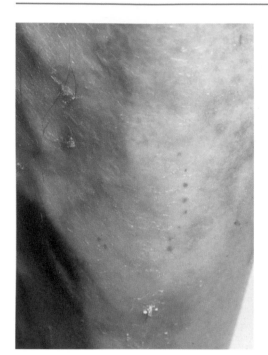

Diabetic dermopathy or 'shin spots' is the most common skin condition associated with diabetes (up to 50% of patients), but it also occurs in a few non-diabetic people (up to 3%). The early lesions are oval, red papules, up to 1 cm in diameter. They slowly become well circumscribed, atrophic, brown and scaly scars. The usual site is the pretibial region, but forearms, thighs and bony prominences may be involved. There is no effective treatment, but the spots tend to resolve over 1–2 years.

Figure 25.1
Diabetic dermopathy.

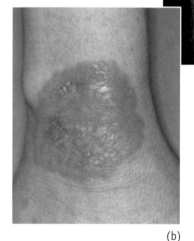

Necrobiosis lipoidica diabeticorum (NDL) is strongly associated with diabetes but rare—occurring in about 0.3% of the diabetic population. The shin is the usual site, where typical chronic lesions are irregularly shaped, indurated plaques with central atrophy. The surface is often shiny with telangiectic vessels crossing a yellowish waxy central area. Ulceration occurs in about 25%. NDL lesions are partially or completely anaesthetic.

Figure 25.2
Necrobiosis lipoidica diabeticorum (NLD). (a) A typical lesion on the front of the shin, with a small satellite lesion below the main area. (b) Necrobiosis at an unusual site on the dorsum of the wrist. Note the typical yellow, atrophic appearance with telangiectasia.

(a)

(b)

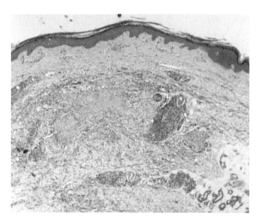

Histologically, NDL lesions show hyaline degeneration of collagen ('necrobiosis'), surrounded by fibrosis and with a diffuse histiocytic infiltrate. The treatment is unsatisfactory, with no response to improved glycaemic control. Corticosteroids may improve early NDL but should not be used in chronic atrophic lesions. Cosmetic camouflage seems the best option in most cases.

Figure 25.3
Histological features of NLD showing degeneration of collagen ('necrobiosis'), associated with fibrosis and a histiocytic infiltrate. Haematoxylin and eosin stain ×40.

HANDBOOK OF DIABETES *2ND EDITION*

The skin is generally thickened by diabetes, probably in large part due to glycation of dermal collagen and cross-linking to form advanced glycation end products and 'browning'. Usually this is clinically insignificant but thickening over the dorsum of the fingers and 'Garrod's knuckle pads' can lead to stiff and painful fingers.

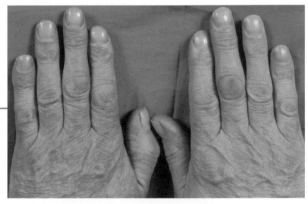

Figure 25.4
Diabetic hand syndrome. Garrod's knuckle pads in a patient with type 1 diabetes. Note thickening of the skin, particularly over the metacarpophalangeal and interphalangeal joints.

In a minority, skin thickening can lead to Dupuytren's contracture and trigger finger.

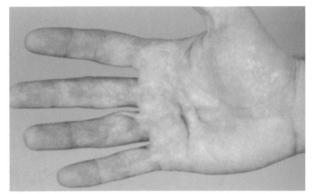

Figure 25.5
Dupuytren's contracture.

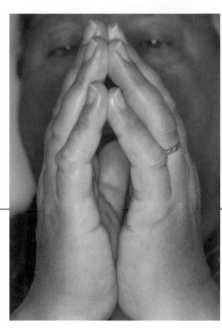

A typical sign of the 'diabetic hand syndrome' or cheiroarthropathy is the 'prayer sign', where limited joint mobility due to thick, tight and waxy skin does not allow the patient to press both hands together.

Figure 25.6
The 'prayer sign'.

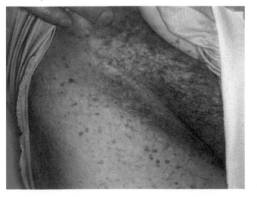

Acanthosis nigricans is a hyperpigmented velvety overgrowth of the epidermis, usually in the flexural areas of the axilla, groin and neck. It is associated with various causes of insulin resistance (such as genetic and autoimmune insulin receptor defects), possibly because raised circulating insulin levels act on insulin-like growth factor-1 (IGF-1) receptors in the skin to stimulate growth.

Figure 25.7
Acanthosis nigricans.

A number of skin problems are associated with long-standing diabetes, including bacterial infections (e.g. boils and sepsis due to *Staphylococcus aureus*), *Candida albicans* infections (e.g. vulvovaginitis, balanitis, intertrigo and chronic paronychia), tinea (dermatophyte infections), neuropathic and ischaemic foot ulcers, and dry skin due to decreased sweating with autonomic neuropathy.

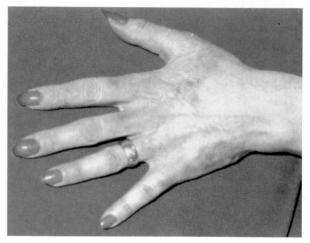

Figure 25.8
Skin infections in diabetic patients. Tinea manum showing characteristic erythematous, scaly margin.

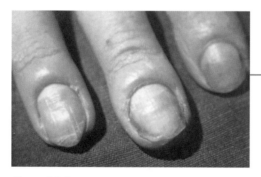

Figure 25.9
Chronic paronychia.

Chronic paronychia presents with swelling and erythema around the nail folds, with a discharge. Severe involvement may produce oncholysis. Treatment is by exclusion of water and antifungal drugs; systemic drugs such as oral fluconazole, rather than topical administrations, may be necessary.

Cutaneous side-effects of antidiabetic drugs include insulin lipoatrophy and lipohypertrophy (see Management of type 1 Diabetes, pp. 80–1), and localised and systemic allergic reactions such as urticaria and pruritus. Skin reactions from sulphonylurea drugs are more frequent with first-generation agents such as cholorpropamide. Reactions include maculopapular rashes and erythema multiforme. The severe form of this is Stevens–Johnson syndrome with typical target lesions, and blistering ulceration which can involve the mouth and eyes. Chlorpropamide also causes a facial flush after drinking alcohol.

(a)

Figure 25.10
Stevens–Johnson syndrome, showing typical 'target' lesions of (a) erythema multiforme and (b) mouth ulceration. Ocular involvement is common and can cause blindness; ophthalmological opinion must always be sought.

(b)

Chapter 26

Psychological and psychiatric problems in diabetes

Diabetic group	Psychological problem
Children and adolescents at onset of diabetes (little known about adults with recent-onset diabetes)	Temporary adjustment disorder — somatic complaints, social withdrawal, sleeping disorder, anxiety, depression
Older adults with established diabetes, especially when hospitalised	Higher frequency of depression (but comparable to other chronic illnesses)
Patients with macrovascular disease and proliferative retinopathy	Depression, poor quality of life, psychological distress

Figure 26.1
Psychological problems that can affect the diabetic person.

Particular groups of diabetic patients are at risk of different psychological problems. In general, children and adolescents are surprisingly free of psychopathology, though psychological stress appears to increase in adulthood. Amongst the problems are adjustment disorders at the onset of diabetes (e.g. sleep disorders, anxiety, social withdrawal); and a higher frequency of psychological stress, including depression, occurs in established diabetes, particularly in hospitalised patients and those with macrovascular disease and sight-threatening retinopathy.

Diabetic group	Psychological group
Children with repeated hypoglycaemia	Mild impairment of cognitive functioning — visuospatial/verbal defects
Adults with hypoglycaemia	Uncertain effects

Figure 26.2 Hypoglycaemia and cognitive function in diabetes.

Mildly impaired cognitive function (e.g. lack of concentration, learning and memory problems) occurs in children with early-onset diabetes, who are especially vulnerable to repeated hypoglycaemia, presumably the influence of hypoglycaemia on the developing nervous system. The psychological effects of repeated hypoglycaemia in adults with diabetes is less certain, probably there is little or no damage.

Diabetic group	Psychological group
Later-onset children/adolescents	Verbal IQ and academic achievement lowered
Adults with chronic hyperglycaemia	Defects in psychomotor tasks, attention, and learning

Figure 26.3 Psychological disorders in older children and adults with diabetes.

Lowered academic achievement has been noted in children and adolescents with later-onset diabetes, not specifically related to metabolic control but more likely due to disrupted education as the result of absences from school and psychosocial problems within the family. In older adults with type 2 diabetes, defects occur in psychomotor tasks, attention, learning and memory which are related to chronic hyperglycaemia. Improved control of diabetes also improves learning and memory in these patients.

The commonest psychiatric disorder in diabetes is depression, which can occur with or without anxiety. Those with chronic complications are particularly at risk. The features of moderate or severe depression should be recognised by diabetologists, though cases are often missed in the setting of a busy diabetic clinic.

Presence of depressed morale or loss of interest and pleasure (for over 2 weeks)
Feelings of worthlessness, guilt or self-blame
Sleep disturbance, fatigue, loss of energy
Loss of appetite, loss of weight
Loss of interests, inactivity
Loss of libido
Inability to concentrate
Marked anxiety
Suicidal thoughts*

*Formal psychiatric referral is also indicated

Figure 26.4
Features of moderate and severe depression suggesting the need for antidepressant drugs.

Treatment of depression

- General measures (diabetic control, sympathetic discussion, specific anxieties, attention to sleep disorders)
- Anti-depressant drugs for non-responders and for moderate/severe depression

Figure 26.5
Treatment of depression.

Depression frequently responds to general measures such as sympathetic discussion, advice on improving glycaemic control and attention to specific causes of anxiety such as fear of blindness, infertility, impotence, amputation etc. Sleep disorders are common and may be helped by regular exercise, avoiding daytime naps, large meals, tobacco, alcohol and caffeine-containing drinks in the evening. Relaxation exercises have been developed to help daytime tension and may also improve control.

Examples

Amitriptyline: sedative: use in agitated or anxious patients

Imipramine: useful in withdrawn or apathetic patients

Dosages

Start at 75 mg/day, increase to 150 mg/day after 1 week

Use lower dosages in elderly patients

Higher dosages (300 mg/day) need specialist supervision

Patients should be told that antidepressant drugs are not addictive
(a common misconception)

Therapeutic effects

Improved sleep and calming effect within a few days

Maximal clinical benefit may take 4–6 weeks

Duration of treatment

Maintain full dosage until symptom-free for 4–6 months

Gradually reduce dosage; do not withdraw abruptly

Some patients require prolonged maintenance treatment

Side-effects (specific contraindications are shown in parentheses)

Dry mouth

Blurred vision (glaucoma)

Hesitancy or retention of urine (prostatism or bladder-neck obstruction)

Tachycardia (arrhythmia, heart block)

Hypotension (autonomic neuropathy)

Sweating

Excessive sedation, with amitriptyline

Late effects developing after 2 weeks include
• Tremor
• Weight gain
• Sexual dysfunction

Moderate or severe depression may require antidepressant drugs. Tricyclic agents are the drugs of first choice. The maximal clinical effect may take 4–6 weeks, and most depression responds over the course of 3–12 months. Treatment should be continued until the patient has been well for 4–6 months, and then gradually reduced. Other antidepressant drugs are tetracyclics (e.g. mianserin), selective serotonin reuptake inhibitors (e.g. fluoxetine), monoamine oxidase inhibitors and lithium salts, but treatment with these agents may be best supervised by a psychiatrist.

Figure 26.6
Tricyclic antidepressant drugs.

Chapter 27
Some intercurrent problems in diabetes

Exercise

In type 1 diabetic patients, glycaemic changes during exercise depend largely on the blood insulin levels and therefore on the type of insulin used and the interval between insulin injection and exercise. For example, hyperinsulinaemia, which occurs when exercise is shortly after the injection of short-acting (regular) insulin, particularly when the site of insulin injection is an exercising limb, causes the blood glucose level to decrease. Hypoinsulinaemia, occurring when exercise is many hours after insulin injection, may cause the blood glucose concentration to rise after exercise.

Blood glucose decreases if:
Hyperinsulinaemia exists during exercise
Exercise is prolonged (>30–60 min) or intensive
Less than 3 h have elapsed since the preceding meal
No extra snacks are taken before or during the exercise
Blood glucose generally remains unchanged if:
Exercise is brief
Plasma insulin concentration is normal
Appropriate snacks are taken before and during exercise
Blood glucose increases if:
Hypoinsulinaemia exists during exercise
Exercise is strenuous
Excessive carbohydrate is taken before or during exercise

Figure 27.1
Factors determining the glycaemic response to acute exercise in type 1 diabetes.

Monitor glycaemia before, during and after exercise as necessary
Avoid hypoglycaemia during exercise by: • Taking 20–40 g extra carbohydrate before and hourly during exercise • Avoiding heavy exercise during peak insulin injection • Using non-exercising sites for insulin injection • Reducing preinjection insulin dosages by 30–50% if necessary
After prolonged exercise, monitor glycaemia and take extra carbohydrate to avoid delayed hypoglycaemia

Figure 27.2
Guidelines for exercise in type 1 diabetes.

Regular exercise which is appropriate for the person's general physical condition and lifestyle is recommended for both type 1 and type 2 diabetic patients. Type 1 diabetic patients can reduce the risk of hypoglycaemia during exercise by following specific guidelines which include close blood glucose monitoring, taking extra carbohydrate before and hourly during exercise, not using exercise sites for injection and sometimes reducing the pre-exercise insulin dose by 30–50%.

| Hypoglycaemia is unlikely during exercise and extra carbohydrate is therefore generally unnecessary |
| Exercise used to reduce weight should be combined with dietary measures |
| Moderate exercise should be part of the daily schedule; heavier exercise (50–70% of VO_{2max}) should be undertaken 3 times/week |
| Include low-intensity warming-up and cooling-down periods |
| Exercise should be appropriate to the person's general physical condition and lifestyle |

Figure 27.3
Guidelines for exercise in type 2 diabetes.

In type 2 diabetes, exercise does not usually cause hypoglycaemia and extra carbohydrate is unnecessary. Exercise accelerates weight loss, increases insulin blood glucose control and lipid profiles, but it should be combined with an appropriate diet and tailored to the individual's capabilities. Everyday moderate exercise is often sustained best, such as 30–60 minutes of walking.

Drugs

Several drugs can induce or worsen hyperglycaemia. Corticosteroids, which are widely prescribed for numerous medical conditions, have the most potent effect. Doses equivalent to prednisolone 30 mg/day or more are especially likely to induce impaired glucose tolerance (IGT) or diabetes in previously normoglycaemic people. Early high-dose oestrogen oral contraceptive pills were likely to cause hyperglycaemia but present combined low-dose or progestogen-only pills have no significant effects on glycaemic control in type 1 diabetes. In type 2 diabetes or in those with a family history of gestational diabetes, oral contraceptives containing the progestogen levonorgestrel should be avoided, and all subjects should be monitored for the onset of hyperglycaemia.

Potentially potent effects	Minor or no effects
Corticosteroids	Oral contraceptives
Oral contraceptives	• Progesterone-only pills
• High-dose oestrogen	Thiazides (low dosage)
• Levonorgestrel in combined pills	Loop diuretics
Thiazide diuretics (conventional dosages)	ACE inhibitors
Beta-2-adrenoreceptor blockers	Calcium-channel blockers
Beta-2-adrenoreceptor agonists	Alpha-1-adrenoreceptor blockers
• Salbutamol	
• Ritodrine	
Others	
• Pentamidine	
• Streptozotocin	
• Diazoxide	
• Cyclosporin	

Figure 27.4
Drugs that cause or exacerbate hyperglycaemia.

Management of corticosteroid-induced diabetes depends largely on the degree of hyperglycaemia. Diet or diet and sulphonylureas are often sufficient, but if significant hyperglycaemia develops, twice daily insulin therapy should be started at a dose of 0.5 U/kg body weight. Type 2 diabetic subjects on high-dose steroids will usually require the addition of sulphonylurea (for diet-treated) or insulin (for tablet-treated patients). For those already on insulin, the dosage may need increasing by 50%, followed by adjustments according to blood glucose values.

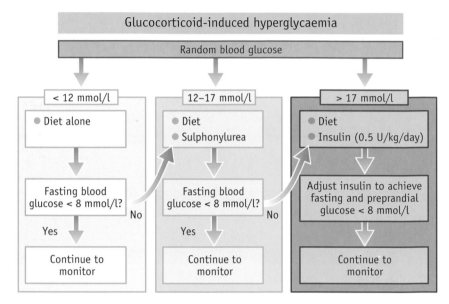

Figure 27.5
Treatment algorithm for glucocorticoid-induced hyperglycaemia.

Several drugs can cause or exacerbate hypoglycaemia. Important examples are alcohol, sulphamethoxazole (combined with trimethoprim in co-trimoxazole) and the numerous drugs that enhance the action of sulphonylureas.

	Decreased clearance	Displaced binding
Drugs that enhance sulphonylureas		
Non-steroidal anti-inflammatory drugs		
Azapropazone	+	+
Phenylbutazone	+	+
Oxyphenbutazone	+	+
Salicylates	+	+
Sulphinpyrazone	+	+
Probenecid	+	+
Sulphonamides	+	+
Monoamine oxidase inhibitors	+	+
Nicoumalone (not warfarin or phenindione)	+	+
Chloramphenicol	+	–
Drugs that interfere with sulphonylureas		
Alcohol		
Rifampicin	Increased hepatic clearance of sulphonylureas	
Chlorpromazine		

Figure 27.6
Drugs that interact with sulphonylureas.

HANDBOOK OF DIABETES 2ND EDITION

Infection

Diabetes is associated with a wide range of bacterial, fungal and viral infections, and diabetes increase the general susceptibility to infection. Hyperglycaemia impairs many of the functions of polymorphs and monocyte/macrophages including chemotaxis, adherence, phagocytosis and intracellular killing of microorganisms. In type 1 diabetes, there may be additional immune defects such as in complement and T-lymphocytes.

Bacterial infections	Fungal infections	Viral infections
Urinary tract	*Genitourinary tract*	Hepatitis B and C
Cystitis	Vulvovaginal candidiasis*	
Emphysematous cystitis*	Invasive candidiasis*	
Pyelonephritis	Renal actinomycosis	
Emphysematous pyelonephritis		
Papillary necrosis*	*Skin and mucosae*	
Perinephric abscess	Mucocutaneous candidiasis	
	Tinea pedis	
Respiratory tract		
Bacterial pneumonia	*Gastrointestinal tract*	
Tuberculosis	Oropharyngeal candidiasis	
	Oesophageal candidiasis	
Gastrointestinal tract		
Periodontal disease	*Respiratory tract*	
Emphysematous cholecystitis	Rhinocerebral mucormycosis*	
	Pulmonary mucormycosis*	
Soft tissues and bone		
Necrotizing fasciitis*	*Central nervous system*	
Necrotizing (malignant) otis externa	Fungal meningitides	
Infected foot ulcers*		
Osteomyelitis		
Rare bacteria		
Enterococcal meningitis		
Meliodosis		
Pyomyositis		

Figure 27.7
Infections associated with diabetes.
*Strong associations with diabetes.

Infection is the major cause of hyperglycaemic crisis in diabetic patients, worsening control or sometimes precipitating ketoacidosis (the commonest cause). Management of diabetes during infection should include careful blood glucose monitoring, maintenance of fluid intake and often increases in the dosages of oral agents or insulin so as to regain glycaemic control. Those on oral agents may need transferring to insulin. Inpatient management of severely ill patients may include intravenous insulin and fluids.

Outpatients

Monitor blood glucose at least 4-hourly
Increase insulin dosage to cover persistent hyperglycaemia
Maintain high fluid intake (low-sugar drinks)
Make and maintain contact wih medical team (ideally the specialist diabetes team)
Seek help immediately if:
• Vomiting develops
• Hyper- or hypoglycaemia develop

Inpatients

Monitor blood glucose at least 4-hourly
Increase insulin dosage to cover hyperglycaemia
• Consider intravenous insulin (e.g. GKI regimen)
Consider insulin treatment in patients taking oral agents
Maintain hydration
• Use intravenous fluids if necessary

Figure 27.8
Control of diabetes during intercurrent infection. GKI, glucose–potassium–insulin infusion (see Figs 27.10 and 27.11).

Surgery

Surgical stress stimulates secretion of counterregulatory hormones such as cortisol and catecholamines, and inhibits insulin secretion. In insulin-deficient diabetic patients, this may cause dangerous hyperglycaemia and ketosis. In general, this is more pronounced in type 1 diabetes. Hypoglycaemia is the other major risk of surgery in diabetic subjects. Safety and simplicity are the guiding principles of diabetes management during surgery. After preoperative assessment to confirm fitness for anaesthesia, optimisation of control, and liaison with the surgical and anaesthetic teams, management plans will depend on whether or not the patient is insulin treated and on the nature and duration of surgery.

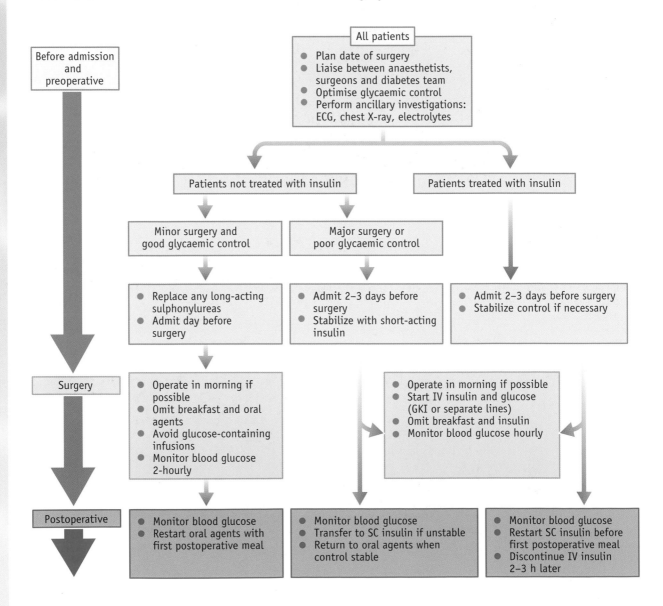

Figure 27.9

Management protocols for surgery in diabetic patients. GKI, glucose–potassium–insulin infusion (see Figs 27.10 and 27.11).

In type 2 diabetic patients, long-acting sulphonylureas should be changed to short-acting agents some days before surgery. Well-controlled patients undergoing minor surgery can omit drugs on the morning of the operation and need close blood glucose monitoring during the perioperative period. In all type 1 patients and for major surgery in type 2 patients, a glucose–potassium–insulin (GKI) infusion is needed to maintain metabolic control.

---

1 Ensure satisfactory preoperative control. Operate in morning if possible

2 Liaise with anaesthetist

3 Omit breakfast, and insulin or oral hypoglycaemic drug, on morning of surgery

4 Non-insulin-treated diabetic patients, having non-major surgery, need observation only. Chart 2-hourly glucose reagent strips on day of surgery. Patients taking oral hypoglycaemic drugs can restart these with next meal

5 'GKI' is used in all other cases, i.e. (a) all insulin–treated diabetic patients, and (b) major surgery in non-insulin-treated diabetic patients

(i) At 0800–0900 on morning of surgery, start GKI infusion:
500 ml 10% dextrose
+ 15 U short-acting insulin   Infuse 5-hourly
+ 10 mmol KCl   (100 ml/h)

(ii) Check blood glucose 2-hourly initially and aim for 6–11 mmol/l
  • If > 11 mmol/l, change to GKI with 20 U insulin
  • If < 6 mmol/, change to GKI with 10 U insulin
Continue to adjust as necessary

(iii) Continue GKI until patients eat, then revert to usual treatment. If GKI is prolonged (> 24 h), check electrolytes daily for possible sodium or potassium abnormalities

Figure 27.10
A simple protocol for managing patients with type 1 or type 2 diabetes undergoing surgery. These guidelines are suitable for use by junior hospital staff with limited specialist experience of diabetes.

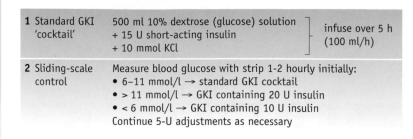

1 Standard GKI 'cocktail'	500 ml 10% dextrose (glucose) solution + 15 U short-acting insulin + 10 mmol KCl	infuse over 5 h (100 ml/h)
2 Sliding-scale control	Measure blood glucose with strip 1-2 hourly initially: • 6–11 mmol/l → standard GKI cocktail • > 11 mmol/l → GKI containing 20 U insulin • < 6 mmol/l → GKI containing 10 U insulin Continue 5-U adjustments as necessary	

Figure 27.11
The glucose–potassium–insulin or GKI system.

A simple 'GKI' regimen consists of continuous intravenous infusion (100 ml/h) of 10% dextrose to which insulin and potassium have been added. To a 500 ml bag of dextrose, 15 units of short-acting insulin and 10 mmol potassium chloride are added and infused over 5 hours. Blood glucose should be monitored every 1–2 hours. Though alterations to the standard mixture are not often needed, in the event of hyper- or hypoglycaemia or electrolyte disturbance, new bags may be used with different insulin or potassium additions.

Chapter 28
Pregnancy and diabetes

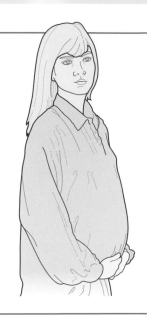

In women with pre-existing diabetes, glycaemic control worsens during pregnancy and insulin requirements increase in type 1 diabetes; ketoacidosis may also develop. This is because pregnancy induces insulin resistance through the diabetogenic effects of placental hormones and progesterone. Insulin resistance-induced hyperglycaemia and enhanced lipolysis in the non-diabetic woman is probably favourable as it encourages nutrient transfer to the growing fetus.

Figure 28.1
Pregnant diabetic woman: control worsens in pregnancy.

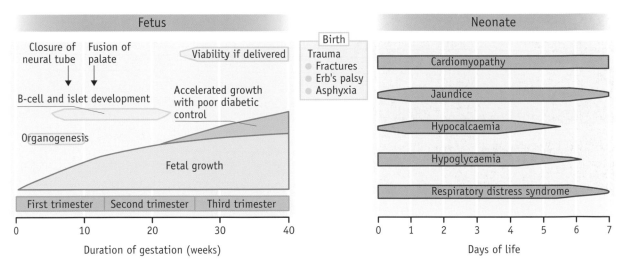

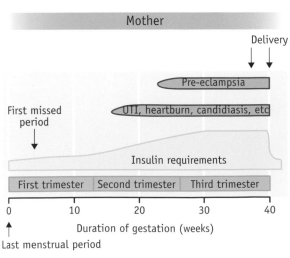

Maternal diabetes influences many aspects of pregnancy, with effects on the fetus, the neonate and the mother. The fetus is adversely affected by malformations, accelerated and inappropriate growth (macrosomia) and altered islet cell development (increased insulin secretion). Though perinatal mortality has fallen, the stillbirth rate remains at about four times that of the non-diabetic population.

Figure 28.2
Impact of maternal diabetes on the fetus and neonate and the mother. UTI, urinary tract infection.

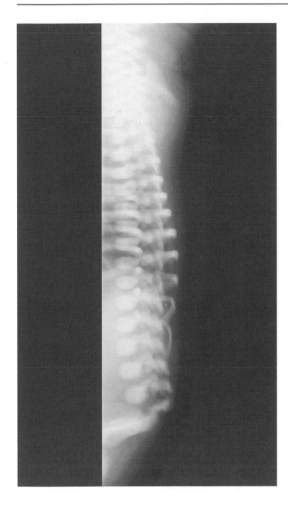

Figure 28.3
Radiograph of the fetus of a diabetic mother, showing sacral agenesis (the caudal regression syndrome).

Diabetes is teratogenic, particularly in the first 8 weeks' gestation when the major organs are forming. Defects include anencephaly, spina bifida, great vessel abnormalities and sacral agenesis. The malformation rate is related to the degree of hyperglycaemia (about 30% in poorly controlled patients) but tight control can probably reduce the rate.

Accelerated fetal growth, leading to macrosomic, large-for-gestational age infants, is due to enhanced delivery of glucose and other nutrients from the mother to the fetus. This stimulates the islets and induces fetal hyperinsulinaemia which promotes abdominal fat deposition, skeletal growth and organomegaly. Complications of these babies include birth trauma and neonatal hypoglycaemia and hypocalcaemia. Poor glycaemic control also leads to impaired production of lung surfactant and risk of respiratory distress syndrome in the neonate.

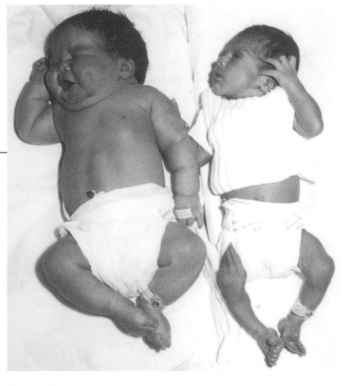

Figure 28.4
Left: a macrosomic baby born to a diabetic mother. Right: a normal baby born to a non-diabetic mother.

Understanding the risks

Perinatal mortality
Congenital anomalies
Maternal mortality
Diabetic complications in pregnancy
Obstetric complications
Inheritance of diabetes in offspring

What a diabetic pregnancy involves

Frequent antenatal visits and close supervision
Strict blood glucose control (home blood
glucose monitoring, optimised insulin regimen)
Stop smoking and drinking alcohol
Appropriate diet

Other advice

Folic acid supplementation
Contraception

Management of pregnancy in women with diabetes begins with pre-conception advice and counselling, which includes explanation of the risks of pregnancy, and the requirements for successful pregnancy (such as frequent clinic visits beginning as soon as possible after conception, optimised metabolic control, stopping smoking and drinking alcohol, and a folate-rich and supplemented diet).

Figure 28.5
Prepregnancy counselling.

First trimester management of pregnancy in type 1 diabetes includes optimisation of control, aiming for a fasting blood glucose <5 mmol/l and postprandial peaks <7 mmol/l, and screening for complications. Pregnancy can worsen renal function in those with established nephropathy—increased proteinuria and hypertension are common. Hypertension should be controlled with non-teratogenic agents such as methyldopa and/or nifedipine (ACE inhibitors are contraindicated). Retinopathy may deteriorate rapidly, especially when control is suddenly improved; early prophylactic photocoagulation may be necessary in certain high-risk cases. Occult ischaemic heart disease should be sought by resting or exercise ECG tests. Myocardial infarction in pregnant diabetic women carries high maternal and fetal mortality.

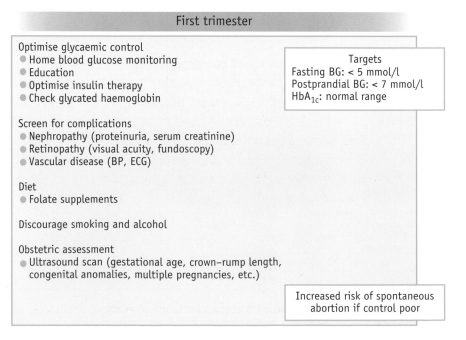

First trimester

Optimise glycaemic control
● Home blood glucose monitoring
● Education
● Optimise insulin therapy
● Check glycated haemoglobin

Screen for complications
● Nephropathy (proteinuria, serum creatinine)
● Retinopathy (visual acuity, fundoscopy)
● Vascular disease (BP, ECG)

Diet
● Folate supplements

Discourage smoking and alcohol

Obstetric assessment
● Ultrasound scan (gestational age, crown–rump length,
  congenital anomalies, multiple pregnancies, etc.)

Targets
Fasting BG: < 5 mmol/l
Postprandial BG: < 7 mmol/l
HbA$_{1c}$: normal range

Increased risk of spontaneous
abortion if control poor

Figure 28.6
First trimester management of diabetic pregnancy.

Second trimester

Monitor glycaemic control
- Home blood glucose monitoring
- Serum fructosamine
- Increased insulin dosage usual

Monitor and treat complications
- Hypertension: methyldopa, nifedipine
- Retinopathy: photocoagulation

Fetal monitoring
- Ultrasound
    - 18–24 weeks: major malformations
    - 20–24 weeks: fetal heart examination
    - 26 weeks onwards: growth and liquor volume

Obstetric assessment, check for complications
- Pre-eclampsia
- Polyhydramnios
- Urinary tract infections
- Vaginal candidiasis
- Carpal tunnel syndrome
- Reflux: oesophagitis

Third trimester

Monitor glycaemic control
- Insulin dose increases to 34–36 weeks, then plateau and small decline

Monitor fetal growth
- Frequent ultrasound scans for macrosomia (abdominal; head circumference) and liquor volume

Maternal complications
- Pre-eclampsia
- Preterm labour

Obstetric assessment includes regular ultrasound scanning for gestational age, detecting major malformations, monitoring fetal growth and macrosomia and for assessing the volume of amniotic fluid. The complications of diabetic pregnancy include pre-eclampsia (hypertension, proteinuria, oedema and fetal compromise), polyhydramnios, urinary tract infections, vaginal candidiasis, carpal tunnel syndrome, reflux oesphagitis and pre-term labour.

Figure 28.7
Second and third trimester management of diabetic pregnancy.

10% dextrose

Drip-counter

100 ml/h

Vein

Soluble insulin
50 U in 50 ml saline

Syringe-driver pump
Titrate rate from hourly blood glucose measurement

During labour, diabetes should be controlled by continuous intravenous infusions of insulin (typically 2–4 U/h) and glucose. After delivery, insulin requirements return rapidly to pre-pregnancy values and insulin should be reduced to avoid hypoglycaemia. Elective Caesarian section is indicated if mechanical problems with vaginal delivery are anticipated (e.g. malpresentation, disproportion), for fetal compromise and severe pre-eclampsia.

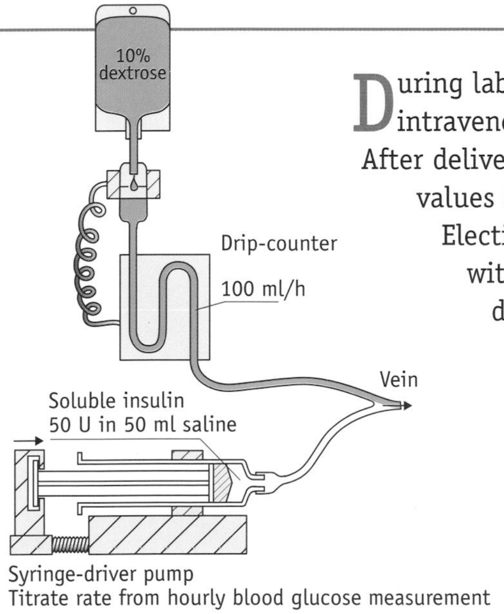

Figure 28.8
Intravenous insulin/glucose infusion system for controlling diabetes during labour.

Management of pregnancy in type 2 diabetes is the same as for type 1 diabetes. In general, women should change insulin before conception or early in the first trimester. Oral hypoglycaemic agents are unlikely to achieve sufficiently good control and cross the placenta, aggravate hyperinsulinaemia (in the case of sulphonylureas) and, though the evidence is conflicting, are potentially teratogenic.

Gestational diabetes is glucose intolerance that is first recognised in pregnancy. Although no diagnostic criteria are agreed, the WHO definition—plasma glucose concentration exceeding 7.8 mmol/l 2 hours after 75 g oral glucose is becoming increasingly used. Risk factors for gestational diabetes include obesity, a family history of type 2 diabetes and gestational diabetes, and a macrosomic infant, stillbirth or neonatal death during a previous pregnancy. The implications and treatment of gestational diabetes are controversial but management should probably be as for established diabetes, and 10–30% require insulin treatment. Diabetes resolves after delivery but is likely to recur in subsequent pregnancies, and the lifetime risk of developing type 2 diabetes is about 30%.

Special features of pregnancy in type 2 diabetes

- In populations where frequency of type 2 diabetes is high (e.g. ethnic minorities), can be more common than pregnancy in type 1 diabetes
- Patients older, more obese than pregnant type 1 diabetic women
- Maternal hypertension more common
- Later presentation
- High rate of fetal loss

Figure 28.9
Special features of pregnancy in type 2 diabetes.

Chapter 29
Diabetes in children

Polyuria, including nocturia and incontinence
Thirst and polydipsia
Weight loss
Growth failure (falling below height and weight centiles)
Increased appetite, especially for carbohydrate-rich foods
Abdominal pains and vomiting
Blurred vision
Muscle cramps
Infections
• Boils, urinary tract infections
• Genital or perineal candidiasis
Behaviour disturbance, poor school performance
Inability to concentrate
Tiredness, lack of energy
Ketoacidosis
• Acidotic (Kussmaul) breathing
• Protracted vomiting
• Dehydration and postural hypotension
• Disturbance of consciousness
• Coma

Diabetes in children is a common and important problem. Over 95% of cases are due to type 1 diabetes, which has a peak age of onset at 12 years. Rare causes of diabetes in childhood include maturity-onset diabetes of the young and various genetic syndromes. The presentation commonly includes nocturia and incontinence, thirst, weight loss and growth failure, general malaise, abdominal pain and vomiting, poor performance or behavioural problems at school and infections.

Figure 29.1
Presenting symptoms of type 1 diabetes in childhood.

With the support of home visits, most newly presenting children with diabetes who are not ketoacidotic need only a short hospital admission (1–2 days) to begin insulin treatment and learn 'first aid' knowledge of diabetes. Fuller education and dietary instruction can be given over the following weeks and months. Initial insulin dosages average 0.5 U/kg/day but are very variable. Most eventually need twice daily insulin injections—premixed biphasic formulations and pen administration are helpful. After initial stabilisation, many show a 'honeymoon period' with a marked fall in the insulin dose for a few months. This is due to a transient improvement in residual B-cell function.

Figure 29.2
Child learning insulin injection.

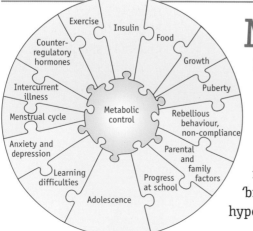

Figure 29.3
Some factors suggested to influence blood glucose control in children with diabetes mellitus.

Metabolic control in children and adolescents with diabetes is influenced by many physiological and psychological factors. Long-term compliance presents many difficulties; omission of insulin and dietary indiscretion are common causes of poor metabolic control. Normal adolescent behaviour encompasses rebellion and experimentation with problems at home or school, but most cope well with their diabetes and only a few suffer from the extreme metabolic chaos termed 'brittle diabetes'—where recurrent ketoacidosis and/or hypoglycaemia disrupt life.

Diabetic ketoacidosis in childhood still carries a high morbidity and mortality. Important causes include intercurrent infection, omission of insulin and poor diabetic education. Treatment demands urgent admission to hospital. Accurate and controlled intravenous fluid replacement is essential—isotonic saline should be given initially, changing to 5% dextrose/saline when blood glucose has fallen to 10 mmol/l. A scheme for fluid administration based on fluid deficit and the normal fluid intake should be followed.

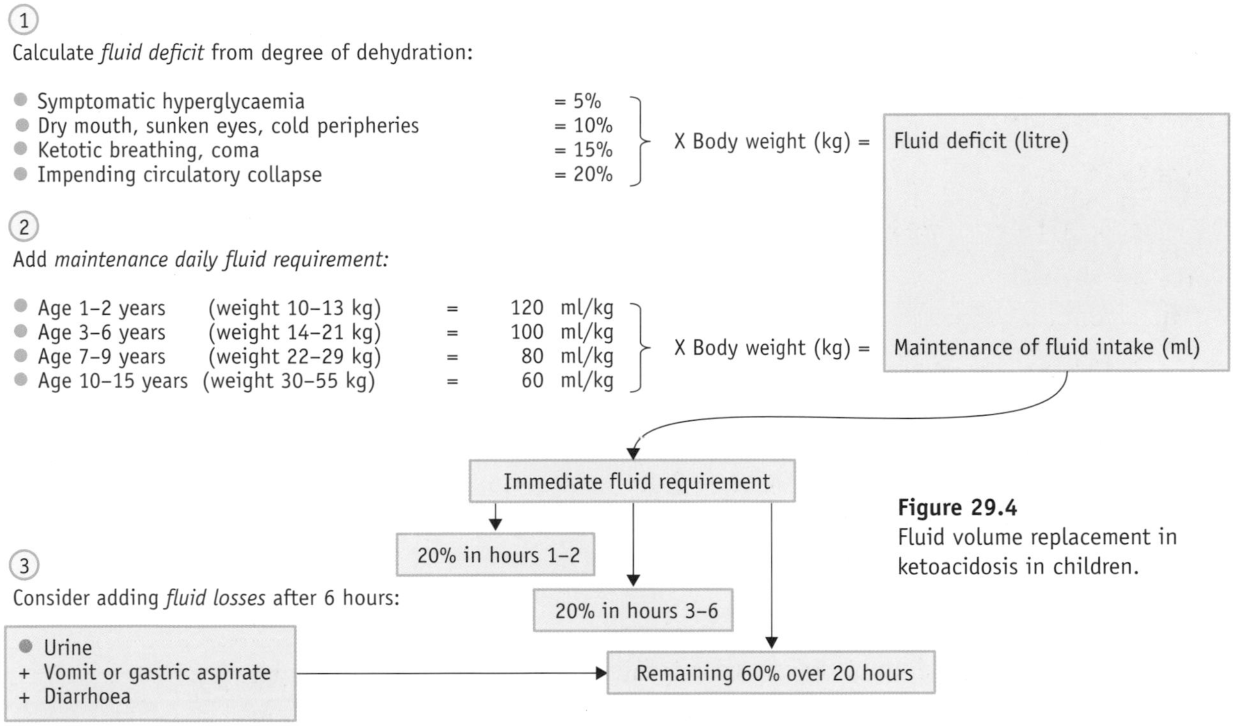

(1)

Calculate *fluid deficit* from degree of dehydration:

- Symptomatic hyperglycaemia = 5%
- Dry mouth, sunken eyes, cold peripheries = 10%
- Ketotic breathing, coma = 15%
- Impending circulatory collapse = 20%

X Body weight (kg) = Fluid deficit (litre)

(2)

Add *maintenance daily fluid requirement*:

- Age 1–2 years   (weight 10–13 kg) = 120 ml/kg
- Age 3–6 years   (weight 14–21 kg) = 100 ml/kg
- Age 7–9 years   (weight 22–29 kg) = 80 ml/kg
- Age 10–15 years (weight 30–55 kg) = 60 ml/kg

X Body weight (kg) = Maintenance of fluid intake (ml)

Immediate fluid requirement

20% in hours 1–2

20% in hours 3–6

(3)

Consider adding *fluid losses* after 6 hours:

- Urine
+ Vomit or gastric aspirate
+ Diarrhoea

Remaining 60% over 20 hours

Figure 29.4
Fluid volume replacement in ketoacidosis in children.

Urgent hospital admission
Fluid replacement
- Volumes
- Isotonic saline; dextrose-saline when blood glucose < 10 mmol/l
- Consider bicarbonate if arterial blood pH < 7.0
- Consider plasma or plasma expander (25 ml/kg) initially if severe hypotension and coma
Potassium replacement
- Generally 20 mmol/l intravenous fluid
- Adjust according to plasma potassium (for electrocardiogram)
Insulin replacement
- Continuous intravenous infusion, initially 0.1 U/kg/h
- Adjust by blood glucose monitoring
Other measures
- Blood glucose monitoring, hourly until stable
- Fluid balance monitoring
- Plasma urea and electrolytes monitoring, 3-hourly until stable
- Arterial blood gases and pH monitoring if acidotic or hypoxaemic
- Consider oxygen; review need for intubation and ventilation
- Electrocardiogram monitoring, if arrhythmias or electrolyte disturbances develop
- Nasogastric intubation, if persistent vomiting or gastric stasis occurs
- Urinary catheterization, if retention or apparent oliguria develops
- If cerebral oedema suspected:
  Avoid fluid overload and use of hypotonic solutions
  Consider intravenous mannitol or dexamethasone

Insulin is best given by continuous intravenous infusion at an initial rate of 0.1 U/kg/h. Potassium generally should be added at the rate of 20 mmol/l of intravenous fluid.

Figure 29.5
Management of diabetic ketoacidosis in children.

Cerebral oedema is the major cause of death in ketoacidosis in childhood. It leads to herniation of the brain stem and cerebellar tonsils into the foramen magnum and respiratory arrest. The pathogenesis is unclear, perhaps involving rapid changes in blood osmolality during over-rapid delivery of fluid or insulin. Clinically, there is headache, depressed consciousness and sometimes papilloedema. A CT scan or MRI confirm the diagnosis. Intravenous mannitol or dexamethazone, given immediately, sometimes reduce intracranial pressure.

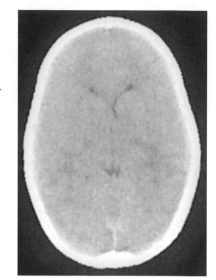

Figure 29.6
CT scan of the brain of a child with diabetic ketoacidosis complicated by cerebral oedema, showing swelling of the brain substance with compression of the lateral ventricles.

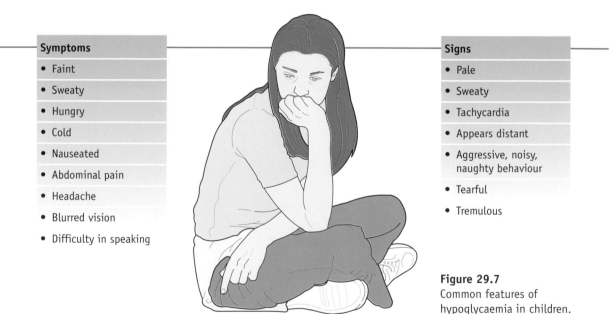

Symptoms	Signs
• Faint	• Pale
• Sweaty	• Sweaty
• Hungry	• Tachycardia
• Cold	• Appears distant
• Nauseated	• Aggressive, noisy, naughty behaviour
• Abdominal pain	• Tearful
• Headache	• Tremulous
• Blurred vision	
• Difficulty in speaking	

Figure 29.7
Common features of hypoglycaemia in children.

Hypoglycaemia is common in diabetic children, often following unusual exercise, a missed meal or an injection error. It is the aspect of diabetes most feared by patients and families. The symptoms vary considerably and include faintness, hunger, sweating, irritability and aggressive or naughty behaviour. Treatment is similar to that in adults with diabetes—oral carbohydrate, or glucagon by intramuscular or deep subcutaneous injection if consciousness is impaired. Those who are semiconscious, comatose, having seizures or do not recover within a few minutes should be admitted urgently to hospital and given intravenous glucose (50–100 ml 50% dextrose, followed if necessary by 10% dextrose infused at 100 ml/h until consciousness is regained or blood glucose is no longer falling).

Chapter 30
Diabetes in the elderly

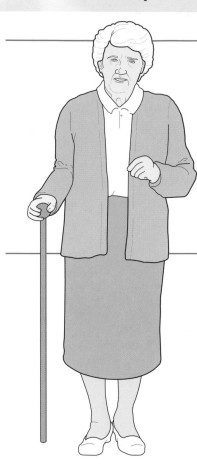

Figure 30.1
Elderly person: diabetes and IGT are common.

Type 2 diabetes and impaired glucose tolerance are common in elderly people. Each affect about 10–20% of subjects over the age of 65 years in many Western countries. The prevalence of diabetes in elderly people is increasing, perhaps because obesity is more frequent or because people with diabetes are surviving longer.

Presentation of diabetes in the elderly
• Symptoms often non-specific (lassitude, incontinence, falls,etc)
• May present with cardiovascular disease
• Myocardial infarction may be silent

Figure 30.2
Presentation of diabetes in the elderly.

Diabetic symptoms in elderly people are often non-specific and vague, such as lassitude, change in mental state or urinary incontinence. Many present with cardiovascular disease (CVD), which in old age may be present with atypical symptoms such as painless myocardial infarction, manifesting instead as cardiac failure, lassitude or falls. Lower-limb ischaemia can occur without claudication, even presenting first as gangrene.

Elderly diabetic people require treatment mainly to alleviate symptoms and reduce the risk of hyperglycaemic crises. Strict glycaemic control regimes may not always be appropriate. Some key points about diabetes treatment in the elderly are: diets are rarely successful in producing weight loss in this group and may be unjustifiably burdensome in the frail; shorter-acting sulphonylureas such as gliclazide are preferred because of the likelihood in the elderly of impaired renal function and other factors that increase the risk of hypoglycaemia; metformin is best avoided because of its increased tendency to lactic acidosis; simple insulin regimens are appropriate but the practical difficulties of administration can limit their use; the general hazards of drug treatment in the elderly include the possibility of multiple drug interactions, non-compliance and inappropriate drug prescribing.

Diabetes in the elderly
• Diet often unsuccessful
• Use short-acting sulphonylureas
• Avoid metformin
• Use simple insulin regimens
• Note drug hazards in the elderly

Figure 30.3
Diabetes in the elderly: treatment points.

HANDBOOK OF DIABETES 2ND EDITION

Chapter 31
Diabetes and lifestyle

Driving

The main problems for diabetic drivers are hypoglycaemia and visual impairment from cataract or retinopathy. Mechanical difficulties from peripheral neuropathy and peripheral vascular disease or lower limb amputation might also cause problems but can often be surmounted by adapting the vehicles or by automatic transmission. There are therefore several reasons why diabetic subjects should cease driving, including recurrent, severe hypoglycaemia and impaired awareness of hypoglycaemia, and severely reduced visual acuity.

Newly diagnosed diabetic patients (particularly insulin-treated) should not drive until glycaemic control and vision are safe

Recurrent hypoglycaemia (particularly if severe)

Impaired awareness of hypoglycaemia

Reduced visual acuity (worse than 6/12 on Snellen chart) in both eyes

Sensorimotor peripheral neuropathy (especially with loss of proprioception)

Severe peripheral vascular disease

Figure 31.1
Reasons for diabetic drivers to cease driving.

General advice to the diabetic driver includes the requirements in most countries to declare diabetes to the relevant licensing or regulatory authority and to insurers, measures to avoid hypoglycaemia, and carrying identification stating that you have diabetes.

You have a legal obligation to inform the licensing authority and your motor insurer

Do not drive if your eyesight deteriorates suddenly; take care if night vision is affected if hypoglycaemia develops, stop driving immediately and leave the driver's seat

Keep an emergency supply of glucose in the vehicle

Avoid long journeys without rest periods and meals; check blood glucose at regular intervals

Carry personal identification indicating that you are diabetic in case of road-traffic accidents

Figure 31.2
Advice for diabetic drivers.

HANDBOOK OF DIABETES 2ND EDITION

Vocational driving
Large goods vehicles (LGV) Passenger-carrying vehicles (PCV) Locomotives or underground trains Professional drivers (chauffeurs) Taxi drivers (variable; depends on local authority)
Civil aviation
Commercial pilots; flight engineers Aircrew Air-traffic controllers
National and emergency services
Armed forces (army, navy, air force) Police force Fire brigade or rescue services Merchant navy Prison and security services
Dangerous areas for work
Offshore oil-rig work Moving machinery Incinerator loading Hot-metal areas Work on railway tracks
Work at heights
Overhead linesmen Crane driving Scaffolding/high ladders or platforms

Figure 31.3
Forms of employment from which insulin-treated diabetic people are generally excluded in the UK.

Employment

Diabetic people can and should be encouraged to undertake a wide range of employment. Employment is generally restricted where hypoglycaemia poses a risk to the diabetic worker or to his colleagues or the general public. In most countries, employment is disbarred in the armed forces, civil aviation, emergency services such as fire fighting and in many forms of commercial driving. Many of the restrictions have been established by individual firms or industries, rather than by legislation. Individual assessment is desirable to take into account the type and method of treatment of diabetes.

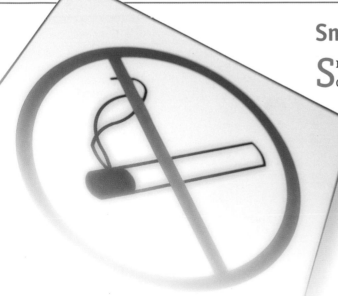

Smoking

Smoking is one of the major avoidable causes of ill health and premature death. Diabetes and smoking interact to produce excess macrovascular disease and mortality. Smoking has also been implicated in the progression of microvascular and other diabetic tissue complications. Strenuous efforts should be made to discourage smoking in diabetic patients, but current anti-smoking policies often fail.

Figure 31.4
Smoking must be discouraged in diabetic people

Travel

Diabetes presents few problems during long-distance travel, though planning for extra supplies, insurance etc. is needed. An extended day during a long Westward plane flight often requires an additional dose of short-acting insulin. Insulin can be kept at warm room temperature (25°C) for at least a month, but it must not be allowed to freeze or be transported in the baggage hold of an aircraft. Potential problems in hot climates include accelerated absorption and action of insulin and damage to neuropathic feet from walking on hot sand.

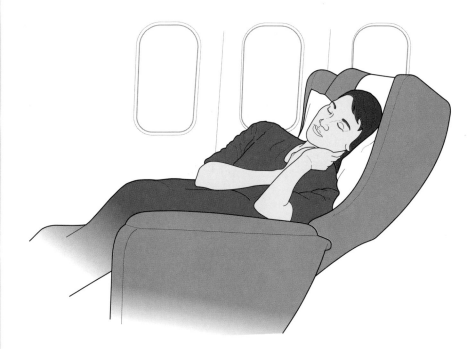

Figure 31.5
Extra insulin may be needed during a long Westward plane flight.

Chapter 32
Organisation of diabetes care

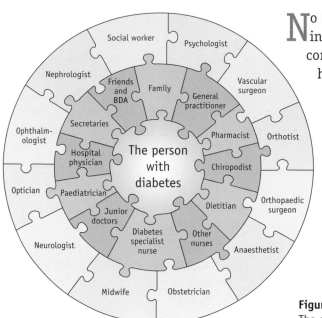

No single person can provide all that is required in diabetes care, and modern management consists of an interacting team involving many hospital specialists (e.g. physicians, ophthalmologists, psychologists, paediatricians, nephrologists, obstetricians, specialist nurses, dietitians, chiropodists etc.), general practitioners and their team, diabetes associations, and the family and friends of the patient.

Figure 32.1
The diabetes care team and how it fits together. BDA, British Diabetes Association (or other national or local association).

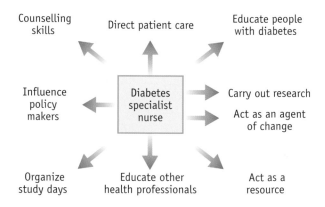

Figure 32.2
The responsibilities of the diabetes specialist nurse.

Diabetes specialist nurses (DSNs) are increasingly playing a major role in diabetes care. Though local needs and facilities govern the exact role of the DSN at a particular centre, there are clear and important responsibilities in education of the patient and staff, counselling, direct patient care, and organisation and policy making in diabetes.

What a diabetic patients' teaching centre should provide
Planning an educational programme for diabetic patients
Group vs. individual diabetic patient education
How to train patients to translate knowledge into action
Use, misuse and abuse of audiovisual aids
Putting a patient on a diet
Starting on insulin
Oral hypoglycaemic agents
Self-monitoring of blood glucose
Motivating the diabetic patient
Foot care
Counselling on late complications
Approaching the parents of a child with diabetes mellitus
Hypoglycaemia
Evaluating diabetes education
Teaching the woman with diabetes about preparing for conception, pregnancy and delivery
Nutrition for the child with diabetes mellitus
Continuing and reinforcing patient education
Educational approaches to the elderly patient with special needs

Diabetic patients should be trained to understand and cope with the everyday demands of diabetes. Effective methods of education include individual and group teaching and computer-based programmes. Interaction and questioning by the patient should be encouraged. Didactic lectures generally fail to alter behaviour. A check list of objectives in diabetes education should be drawn up and agreed with the individual patient. Guidelines for these objectives have been recommended by organisations such as the Diabetes Education Study Group of the EASD (European Association for the Study of Diabetes). Education programmes must be rigorously evaluated to determine outcomes, cost-effectiveness and optimal methods of delivery.

Figure 32.3
Checklist for diabetes education suggested by the Diabetes Education Study Group of the EASD.

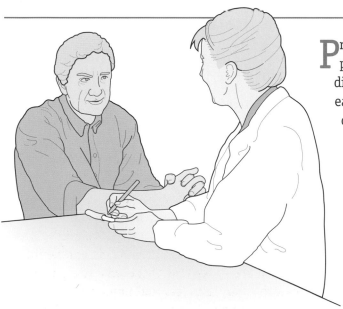

Primary care, administered by general practitioners, has an evolving role in diabetes management. Its advantages include early contact with the patient, and therefore opportunities for screening, diagnosis and prevention. General practitioners provide the long-term medical, psychological, social and family support needed for multi-system diseases such as diabetes. 'Shared care' schemes which integrate hospital and community diabetes care are increasingly popular, and particularly appropriate for patients without significant complications.

Figure 32.4
General practice has an important role in diabetes care.

HANDBOOK OF DIABETES *2ND EDITION*

Uncomplicated diabetic patients may be followed up in general practice at regular intervals. Guidelines for the procedures involved include review of general health, work and school attendance, glycaemic control, diet, tissue complications, diabetes education and whether there is need for referral to the hospital clinic.

Initial visits

Complete examination
- Visual acuity and dilated fundoscopy
- Blood pressure, weight, height, examination for neuropathy

Investigations
- Electrocardiogram

Urinalysis for glucose, protein, ketones, infection and microscopy

Blood for HbA$_1$, creatinine, electrolytes and glucose
- Lipids (may be delayed until blood glucose under control)
- Dietary advice (referral to dietician recommended)
- Start teaching programme (clear explanation of diabetes and its implications)

Frequent visits for education, laboratory tests and contact with the dietician until patient confident in self care and condition stable

Review visits

History
- Patient's perceived problems, general health, hyper/hypoglycaemic symptoms, home monitoring results, days off work/school, diet review

Examination
- Blood pressure, weight

Investigations
- Fasting blood glucose/HbA$_1$, urinalysis for protein

Education
- Continue teaching programme: self-monitoring, dietary advice, foot care, support groups, driving implications, prescription exemption, smoking and exercise

Adjust treatment if necessary

Annual review

Examination
- Blood pressure (lying and standing), weight, injection sites
- Examine for complications, including macroangiopathy
- Foot inspection including pulses and sensation
- Dilated fundoscopy and visual acuity

Investigations
- Urinalysis for glucose, protein, ketones, microscopy and culture
- HbA$_1$, creatinine, electrolytes, glucose and lipids if indicated

Education
- Review educational needs
- Check self-monitoring technique, discuss contraception, preconception and sexual function as appropriate

Reconsider therapy

Consider referral to hospital clinic, dietician, chiropodist and nurse specialist
- Agree management plan with patient for the year, e.g. target weight, HbA$_1$, educational areas

Figure 32.5
Guide for the clinical monitoring of diabetes in general practice.

HANDBOOK OF DIABETES 2ND EDITION

Acknowledgements

Contributors to the *Textbook of Diabetes,* second edition

William Alexander, Kent, UK
Stephanie Amiel, London, UK
Jean-Philippe Assal, Geneva, Switzerland
Clifford Bailey, Birmingham, UK
Stephen Bain, Birmingham, UK
Dennis Barnes, Tunbridge Wells, UK
Anthony Barnett, Birmingham, UK
Peter Barry, Dublin, Ireland
John Betteridge, London, UK
Anne Bishop, London, UK
Michael Bliss, Toronto, Canada
Donatella Bloise, Rome, Italy
Adrian Bone, Brighton, UK
Andrew Boulton, Manchester, UK
David Bowen Jones, Wirral, UK
Jennifer Braimon, Boston, USA
Reinhard Bretzel, Giessen, Germany
Michael Brownlee, New York, USA
Jan Bruining, Rotterdam, Holland
Ken Chiu, Los Angeles, USA
Anne Clark, Oxford, UK
Basil Clarke, Edinburgh, UK
Oscar Crofford, Nashville, USA
Kennedy Cruickshank, Manchester, UK
Anne Dornhorst, London, UK
Jonathan Dowler, London, UK
John Dupré, London, Canada
Michael Edmonds, London, UK
Ole Eshøj, Odense, Denmark
Alberto Falorni, Perugia, Italy
Konrad Federlin, Giessen, Germany
Anne-Marie Felton, London, UK
Robin Ferner, Birmingham, UK
Peter Flatt, Coleraine, UK
Sándor Forgács, Budapest, Hungary
John Forrester, Aberdeen, UK
Alan Foulis, Glasgow, UK
Brian Frier, Edinburgh, UK
Ida Giardino, New York, USA
Geoffrey Gill, Liverpool, UK

Raj Gill, London, UK
Joanna Girling, London, UK
Neil Gittoes, Birmingham, UK
Barry Goldstein, Philadelphia, USA
Rosaire Gray, London, UK
Anders Green, Odense, Denmark
Stephen Greene, Dundee, UK
Anasuya Grenfell, London, UK
Simon Griffin, Cambridge, UK
Leif Groop, Malmö, Sweden
Deirdre Grzebalski, Newcastle upon Tyne, UK
Diane Gwilliam, Brighton, UK
Thomas Ha, Glasgow, UK
Peter Hamilton, London, UK
Andrew Hattersley, Exeter, UK
Bernhard Hering, Giessen, Germany
William Herman, Ann Arbor, USA
Simon Howell, London, UK
James Jackson, Woking, UK
Colin Johnston, Herts, UK
Roland Jung, Dundee, UK
Ron Kahn, Boston, USA
Harry Keen, London, UK
Martin Kendall, Birmingham, UK
Ann-Louise Kinmonth, Cambridge, UK
Roland Klein, Madison, USA
Anthony Knight, Aylesbury, UK
Rachel Knott, Aberdeen, UK
Veikko Koivisto, Helsinki, Finland
Andrew Krentz, Southampton, UK
Andrzej Krolewski, Boston, USA
Yolanta Kruszynska, La Jolla, USA
Michael Lean, Glasgow, UK
Åke Lernmark, Seattle, USA
David Leslie, London, UK
Brigitta Linde, Stockholm, Sweden
Martin Lombard, Liverpool, UK
Ian MacFarlane, Liverpool, UK
Jeffrey Mahon, London, Canada
Aldo Maldonato, Rome, Italy

Eleftheria Maratos-Flier, Boston, USA
David Matthews, Oxford, UK
Teresa McLean, Cambridge, UK
Catherine Mijovic, Birmingham, UK
V. Mohan, Royapettah, India
David Moller, Rahway, USA
Malcolm Nattrass, Birmingham, UK
Ray Newton, Dundee, UK
Peter Nilsson, Lund, Sweden
Paul O'Toole, Liverpool, UK
Alan Permutt, St Louis, USA
Julia Polak, London, UK
G. Premalatha, Royapettah, India
Christopher Ryan, Pittsburgh, USA
Christopher Saudek, Baltimore, USA
Graham Sharpe, Liverpool, UK
Angela Shore, Exeter, UK
Anne Sjølie, Odense, Denmark
Judith Steel, Kirkcaldy, UK
Calvin Stiller, London, Canada
Robert Stout, Belfast, UK
Howard Tager, Chicago, USA (deceased)
Robert Tattersall, Nottingham, UK
Solomon Tesfaye, Sheffield, UK
John Tooke, Exeter, UK
Roberto Trevisan, Padua, Italy
Peter Veld, Rotterdam, Holland
Giancarlo Viberti, London, UK
John Ward, Sheffield, UK
James Warram, Boston, USA
Peter Watkins, London, UK
John Wilding, Liverpool, UK
Greg Wilkinson, Liverpool, UK
Jacqueline Wilkinson, Harrow, UK
Rhys Williams, Leeds, UK
Stephen Wood, Southampton, UK
Hannele Yki-Järvinen, Helsinki, Finland
Ji-Won Yoon, Calgary, Canada
Robert Young, Salford, UK
John Yudkin, London, UK

We are most grateful to the following for supplying illustrations

Professor Michael Berger, Düsseldorf, Germany
Professor S. Bloom, Hammersmith Hospital, London, UK
Dr A. Carty, Royal Liverpool Hospital, Liverpool, UK
Professor H. Carty, Alder Hey Hospital, Liverpool, UK
Eli Lilly and Co, Basingstoke, UK
Dr L.J. Elsas, Emory University, Atlanta, USA
Dr G. Gill, University Hospital Aintree, Liverpool, UK

Dr I. MacFarlane, University Hospital Aintree, Liverpool, UK
Dr H.W. Matthewson, Addenbrooke's Hospital, Cambridge, UK
Dr S. Sandler, University of Uppsala, Sweden
Thomas Fisher Rare Book Library, University of Toronto, Canada
The Wellcome Institute Library, London, UK
The late Professor M. White, University of Hull, UK
Dr J. Verbov, Royal Liverpool Hospital, UK

Figures courtesy of:

1.6 From the World Health Organization Study Group. *Prevention of Diabetes Mellitus*. Technical Report nos 727 and 844. Geneva: World Health Organization, 1994, with permission.

2.1 From the Wellcome Institute Library, London.

2.2 Adapted from Papaspyros S. *The History of Diabetes Mellitus,* 2nd edn. Stuttgart: Thieme, 1964.

2.3 From the Wellcome Institute Library, London.

2.4 From the Wellcome Institute Library, London.

2.5 From the Wellcome Institute Library, London.

2.6 From Bernard C. *Leçons de Physiologie Expérimentale Appliqués à la Médecine.* Paris: Baillière, 1855: 296–313.

2.7 From the Wellcome Institute Library, London.

2.10 From M. Berger, Dusseldorf, Germany.

2.11 From the Thomas Fisher Rare Book Library, University of Toronto, Canada.

2.14 From the Thomas Fisher Rare Book Library, University of Toronto, Canada.

2.17 From the Godfrey Argent Studio, London.

2.18 From the Godfrey Argent Studio, London.

3.6 Adapted from Tattersall R., Gale E. Patient monitoring of blood glucose and refinements of conventional insulin treatment. *Am J Med* 1981; **70**: 77–82.

3.7 Adapted from Paisey R.B. The relationship between blood glycosylated haemoglobin and home capillary blood glucose levels in diabetics. *Diabetologia 1980;* **19**: 31–4.

5.1 Adapted from Songer T. The economic costs of NIDDM. *Diab Metab Rev* 1992; **8**: 389–404 and American Diabetes Association. *Direct and Indirect Costs of Diabetes in the USA in 1992*. Alexandria, VA: American Diabetes Association, 1993.

5.2 From Marks H.H., Krall L.P. Onset, course, prognosis and mortality in diabetes mellitus. In: Marble A., White P. *et al.*, eds. *Joslin's Diabetes Mellitus*, 12th edn. Philadelphia: Lea & Febiger, 1988: 209–54.

6.15 From Lienhard G.E., Slot J.W., James D.E., Mueckler M.M. How cells absorb glucose. *Sci Am* 1992; **266** (1) 34–9. From M. Mueckler and with permission of the Editor of *Scientific American*.

7.1 From Staines A., Bodansky H.J. Lilley H.E.B. *et al*. The epidemiology of diabetes mellitus in the United Kingdom: the Yorkshire Regional Childhood Diabetes Register. *Diabetologia* 1993; **36**: 1282–7.

7.2 After Diabetes Epidemiology Research International Study Group. Preventing insulin-dependent diabetes mellitus: the environmental challenge. *BMJ* 1987; **295**: 479–81. With permission of the Editor of the *British Medical Journal*.

7.3 From Alleyne S.A., Cruickshank J.K., Morrison E. Mortality from diabetes in Jamaica. *Bulletin of PAHO* 1989; **23**: 306–15.

7.4 Data from Sayeed M.A., Khan A.R., Banu A., Hussain M.Z., Ali S.M. Blood pressure and glycaemia status in relation to body mass index in a rural population of Bangladesh. *Bangladesh Med Res Counc Bull* 1994; **20**: 27–35.

7.5 From Scott F.L.V., *Am J Clin Nutr* 1990; **51**: 489–91.

7.17 From S. Sandler, Abstracts of Uppsala Dissertations from the Faculty of Medicine, University of Uppsala, Sweden (1983).

8.2 From Glatthaar C., Welborn T.A., Stenhouse N.S., Garcia-Webb P. Diabetes and impaired glucose tolerance. A prevalence estimate based on the Busselton 1981 survey. *Med J Aust* 1985; **143**: 436–40.

8.3 Adapted from King H., Rewers M., WHO Ad Hoc Diabetes Reporting Group. Global estimates for prevalence of diabetes mellitus and IGT in adults. *Diabetes Care* 1993; **16**: 157–77.

8.4 Data from: Mather H.M., Keen H. The Southall diabetes survey: prevalence of known diabetes in Asians and Europeans. *BMJ* 1985; **291**: 1081–4; Verna N.P.S., Mehta S.P., Madhu S. *et al*. Prevalence of known diabetes in an urban environment: the Darya Ganj diabetes survey. *BMJ* 1986; **293**: 422–3.

8.5 From West K. *Epidemiology of Diabetes and its Vascular Lesions*. Elsevier, 1978.

8.6 Redrawn with permission of the Editors of *Public Health Reports* and *Scandinavian Journal of Clinical Laboratory Investigation*.

8.7 From Meyers J.M., Stunkard A.J. Genetics and human obesity. In: Stunkard A.J., Wadden T.A., eds. *Obesity Theory of Therapy*, 2nd edn. New York: Raven Press, 1993:137–49.

8.9 From Jung R.T. *Colour Atlas of Obesity*. London: Wolfe Medical Publications, 1990.

8.17 From Hosker J.P., Rudenski A.S., Burnett M.A., Mathews D.R., Turner R.C. Similar reduction of first and second-phase B-cell responses at three different glucose levels in type II diabetes and the effect of gliclazide therapy. *Metabolism* 1989; **38**: 767–72.

8.20 From G.M. Reaven, Stanford University School of Medicine, California, USA.

8.21 From Reaven G.M. Role of insulin resistance in human disease. Banting Lecture. *Diabetes* 1988; **37**: 1595–1607.

9.1 From Dr Geoffrey Gill, University Hospital, Aintree, Liverpool, UK.

9.2 From Guy's Hospital, London.

9.3 From Moller D.E., O'Rahilly S. Syndromes of severe insulin resistance. In: Moller D.E., ed. *Insulin Resistance*. Chichester: John Wiley and Sons, 1993: 49–81.

9.4 From L.J. Elsas II, Emory University, Atlanta, GA, USA. From Moller D.E., O'Rahilly S. Syndromes of severe insulin resistance. In: Moller D.E., ed. *Insulin Resistance*. Chichester: John Wiley and Sons, 1993: 49–81.

9.7 From M. White, Royal Liverpool Hospital.

9.11 From A. Carty, Royal Liverpool Hospital, Liverpool.

9.12 From S. Bloom, Royal Postgraduate Medical School, London.

10.2 Adapted from Tattersall R., Gale E. Patient self-monitoring of blood glucose and refinements of conventional insulin treatment. *Am J Med* 1981; **70**: 177–82.

10.7 From Small M., MacRury S., Boal A., Paterson K.R., MacCuish A.C. Comparison of conventional twice daily subcutaneous insulin administration and a multiple injection regimen (using the NovoPen) in insulin-dependent diabetes mellitus. *Diabetes Res* 1988; **8**: 85–9.

10.10 Adapted from Ashby J.P., Frier B.M. Is serum fructosamine a clinically useful test? *Diabet Med* 1988; **5**: 118–21.

11.4 From Eli Lilly and Co.

11.5 From Van Haeften T., Heiling V., Gerich J. Adverse effects of insulin antibodies on postprandial plasma glucose and insulin profiles in diabetic patients without immune insulin resistance: implications for intensive regimens. *Diabetes* 1987; **36**: 305–9.

11.8 From Brange J., Owens D., Kang S., Volund A. Monomeric insulins and their experimental and clinical implications. *Diabetes Care* 1990; **13**: 923–54.

11.9 Modified from Brange J., Owens D., Kang S., Volund A. Monomeric insulins and their experimental and clinical implications. *Diabetes Care* 1990; **13**: 923–54.

11.11 From G. Gill, University Hospital Aintree, Liverpool, with permission of the Editor of *Diabetes Care*.

11.12 From Wilkin T., Keller U., Diaz J.L., Armitage M. Delayed disappearance of human compared to porcine insulin in a patient with insulin autoimmune diabetes. *Res Clin Pract* 1990; **8**: 131–6.

11.15 From Gale E.A.M., Tattersall R.B. Unrecognised nocturnal hypoglycaemia in insulin treated diabetes. *Lancet* 1979; **i**:1049–52

11.16 From Jacobs M.A., Keulen E.T., Kanc K. *et al.* Metabolic efficacy of preprandial administration of Lys(B28), Pro(B29) human insulin analog in IDDM patients. A comparison with human regular insulin during a three-meal test period. *Diabetes Care.* 1997; **20**(8); 1279–86.

11.17 From Home *et al. Diabetes Care* 1998; **21**: 1904–9.

12.5 From Hollander P.A., Elbein S.C., Hirsch I.B. *et al.* Role of orlistat in the treatment of obese patients with type 2 diabetes. A 1-year randomized double-blind study. *Diabetes Care.* 1998; **21**(8): 1288–94.

12.9 From Groop L. Sulfonylureas in NIDDM. *Diabetes Care* 1992; **15**: 737–54.

13.7 From Gareth Williams, University of Liverpool.

14.1 From Pramming S., Thorsteinsson B., Bendtson I., Binder C. Symptomatic hypoglycaemia in 411 Type 1 diabetic patients. *Diabet Med* 1991; **8**: 217–22.

14.4 From The Diabetes Control and Complications Trial Research Group. The effect of intensive treatment of diabetes on the development and progression of long-term complications in insulin-dependent diabetes mellitus. *N Engl J Med* 1993; **329**: 977–86.

14.5 From Pramming S., Thorsteinsson B., Bendtson I., Binder C. Symptomatic hypoglycaemia in 411 Type 1 diabetic patients. *Diabet Med* 1991; **8**: 217–22.

14.6 From Bolli G., De Feo P., Compagnucci P. *et al.* Abnormal glucose counterregulation in insulin-dependent diabetes mellitus. Interaction of anti-insulin antibodies and impaired glucagon and epinephrine secretion. *Diabetes* 1983; **32**: 134–41.

14.7 From Cryer P.E. Iatrogenic hypoglycemia as a cause of hypoglycemia-associated autonomic failure in IDDM. A vicious circle. *Diabetes* 1992; **41**: 255–60.

15.1 From Pirart J. Diabetes mellitus and its degenerative complications: a prospective study of 4400 patients observed between 1947 and 1973. Diabetes Care 1978; **1**: 168–88, 262–61.

15.2 From The Diabetes Control and Complications Trial Research Group. The effect of intensive treatment of diabetes on the development and progression of long-term complications in insulin-dependent diabetes mellitus. *N Engl J Med* 1993; **329**: 977–86.

15.3 From The Diabetes Control and Complications Trial Research Group. The effect of intensive treatment of diabetes on the development and progression of long-term complications in insulin-dependent diabetes mellitus. *N Engl J Med* 1993; **329**: 977–86.

15.4 UK Prospective Diabetes Study (UKPDS) Group. Intensive blood-glucose control with sulphonylureas or insulin compared with conventional treatment and risk of complications in patients with type 2 diabetes (UKPDS 33). *Lancet.* 1998; **352**(9131): 837–53.

16.5 This and other DRS photographs are reproduced by kind permission of the Fundus Photo Reading Center, University of Wisconsin, Madison, USA.

16.11 Adapted from EURODIAB IDDM Complications Study Group. Microvascular and acute complications in IDDM patients: the EURODIAB IDDM Complications Study. *Diabetologia* 1994; **37**: 278–85.

17.1 From A. Morley, Dept of Pathology, Medical School, University of Newcastle upon Tyne.

17.4 Data adapted from Krolewski A.S., Laffel L.M.B., Krolewski M., Quinn M., Warram J.H. Glycosylated hemoglobin and risk of microalbuminuria in patients with insulin-dependent diabetes mellitus. *N Engl J Med* 1995; **332**: 1251–5; Warram J.H., Gearin G., Laffel L., Krolewski A.S. Effect of duration of Type I diabetes on the prevalance of stages of diabetic nephropathy defined by urinary albumin/creatinine ratio. *J Am Soc Nephrol* 1996; **7**: 930–7; Krolewski M., Eggers P., Warram J.H. Magnitude of end-stage renal disease in IDDM: a 35-year follow-up study. *Kidney Int* 1996.

17.7 From Viberti G.C., Hill R.D., Jarrett R.J., Argyropoulos A., Mahmud U., Keen H. Microalbuminuria as a predictor of clinical nephropathy in insulin-dependent diabetes mellitus. *Lancet* 1982; **i**: 1430–2.

17.8 Borch-Johnsen K., Anderson P.K., Deckert T. The effect of proteinuia on relative mortality in type 1 (insulin-dependent) diabetes mellitus. *Diabetologia.* 1989; **28**: 590–6.

17.10 Adapted from Barzilay J., Warram J.H., Bak M., Laffel L.M.B., Canessa M., Krolewski A.S. Predisposition to hypertension: risk factor for nephropathy and hypertension in IDDM. *Kidney Int* 1992; **41**: 723–30.

17.12 From Jones RH, Hayakawa H, MacKay JD, Parsons V, Watkins PJ. Progression of diabetic nephropathy. *Lancet* 1979; **i**: 1105-6.

17.13 From Parving H-H, Andersen A.R, Smidt U.M, Hommel E, Mathiesen E.R, Svendsen P.A. Effect of antihypertensive treatment on kidney function in diabetic nephropathy. *BMJ* 1987; **294**: 1443–7.

18.3 From G. Gill, University Hospital Aintree, Liverpool.

18.7 From Gareth Williams, University of Liverpool.

19.2 From Reaven G.M. Role of insulin resistance in human disease. Banting Lecture. *Diabetes* 1988; **37**: 1595–1607.

20.2 From: Krolewski A.S, Warram J.H, Christlieb A.R, Busick E.J, Kahn C.R. The changing natural history of nephropathy in Type 1 diabetes. *Am J Med* 1985; **78**: 785–94; Krolewski A.S, Warram J.H. Epidemiology and genetics of hypertension in diabetes mellitus. In: Draznin B., Eckel R.H., eds. *Diabetes and Atherosclerosis. Molecular Basis and Clinical Aspects.* New York: Elsevier, 1993: 339–56.

21.2 Data adapted from Vaccaro O., The Multiple Risk Factor Intervention Trial. The 26th annual meeting of the European Diabetes Epidemiology Group, Lund, 1991.

21.4 Adapted from Whitehall Study.

21.6 From Reaven G.M. Role of insulin resistance in human disease. Banting Lecture. *Diabetes* 1988; **37**: 1595–1607.

21.9 From Herlitz J., Malmberg K., Karlson B.W., Ryden L., Hjalmarson A. Mortality and morbidity during a five year follow up of diabetics with myocardial infarction. *Acta Med Scand* 1988; **224**: 31–8.

21.10 Data from Pyörälä *et al.*, University of Kuopio study, Finland.

21.11 Data from Pyörälä *et al.*, University of Kuopio study, Finland.

21.12 From Malmberg K., Ryden L., Efendic S. *et al.* on behalf of the DIGAMI study group. A randomised trial of insulin-glucose infusion followed by subcutaneous insulin treatment in diabetic patients with acute myocardial infarction (Oigami study): effects in mortality at 1 year. *J Am Coll Cardiol* 1995; **26**: 57–65.

22.4 From G. Gill, University Hospital Aintree, Liverpool.

22.7 From Gareth Williams, University of Liverpool.

22.8 From I. MacFarlane, Aintree Hospitals, Liverpool.

23.1 From Bancroft J. *Human Sexuality and its Problems.* Edinburgh: Churchill Livingstone, 1989.

23.3 Adapted from Mersdorf A., Goldsmith P.C. Diederichs W. *et al.* Ultrastructural changes in impotent penile tissue: a comparison of 65 patients. *J Urol* 1991; **145**: 749–58.

23.9 Adapted from Franks S. Polycystic ovary syndrome. *N Engl J Med* 1995; **333**: 853–61 and from Dunaif A., Segal K.R., Futterweit W., Dobrjansky A. Profound peripheral insulin resistance, independent of obesity, in polycystic ovary syndrome. *Diabetes* 1989; **38**: 1165–74.

23.13 From Lawrenson R.A., Newson R.B., Feher M.D., *Practical Diabetes International* 1998; **15**: 71–2.

24.7 From J. Verbov, Royal Liverpool University Hospital.

25.2 From G.V. Gill, University Hospital, Aintree, Liverpool.

25.4 From Dr Geoffrey Gill, University Hospital Aintree, Liverpool, UK.

25.5 From Dr Geoffrey Gill, University Hospital, Aintree, Liverpool, UK.

25.7 From S. Mendelsohn, Countess of Chester Hospital, Chester.

25.10 From S. Mendelsohn, Countess of Chester Hospital, Chester.

28.3 From I. MacFarlane, University Hospital Aintree, Liverpool.

29.5 From H. Carty, Alder Hey Hospital, Liverpool.

31.3 From Waclawski E.R. Employment and diabetes: a survey of the prevalence of diabetic workers known by occupation physicians, and the restrictions placed on diabetic workers in employment. *Diabet Med* 1989; **6**: 16–19.

32.5 From Alberti K.G.M.M, Gries F.A. Management of noninsulin dependent diabetes mellitus in Europe: a consensus view. *Diabet Med* 1988; **5**: 275–81; Patient Services Advisory Committee of the British Diabetic Association. *Recommendations for Diabetes Health Promotion Clinics.* London: British Diabetic Association, 1991; Waine C. *Diabetes in General Practice.* 3. London: Royal College of General Practitioners, 1992.

Index